The Hong Kong Economic Policy Studies Series

HEALTH CARE DELIVERY AND FINANCING:
A MODEL FOR REFORM

T0154858

HEALTH CARE DELIVERY AND FINANCING: A MODEL FOR REFORM

Lok Sang Ho

Published for

The Hong Kong Centre for Economic Research

The Hong Kong Economic Policy Studies Forum

by

City University of Hong Kong Press

First published 1997
Printed in Hong Kong

ISBN 962-937-011-5

Published by
City University of Hong Kong Press
City University of Hong Kong
Tat Chee Avenue, Kowloon, Hong Kong

Internet: http://www.cityu.edu.hk/upress/
E-mail: upress@cityu.edu.hk

The free-style calligraphy on the cover, *jian*, means "health" in Chinese.

Contents

Detailed Chapter Contents vii
Foreword xi
Foreword by the Series Editor xiii
Preface... xv
List of Illustrations xvii

1   Introduction 1
2   The Current Health Care System 19
3   Economic Dimensions of Health Care and Principles
    in Health Policy 43
4   The Available Policy Options 61
5   Recommendations 83
6   Epilogue 99

Appendix A   Notes on Three Surveys................................... 107
Appendix B   Cost Structure in Health Care......................... 117
Appendix C   Statistical Tables of Chapter 2........................ 121
Bibliography.. 135
Index.. 137
About the Author.. 141
About the Series 142

Detailed Chapter Contents

1 Introduction **1**

The Present System under Stress   9
Conclusions   17
Notes   18

2 The Current Health Care System **19**

Introduction   19
The Evaluative Framework   21
    The Perennial Trade-off between Quality,
        Financial Accessibility, and Least Burden   21
Quality of Service   23
Financial Accessibility: Are the Poor Denied Needed Services? 28
    Is Hong Kong's Medical Care System Burdensome?   32
Financial Burden   32
    Public Debate on Burden   35
    Production Efficiency and Consumption Efficiency   36
Autonomy and Freedom of Choice   38
Conclusions   40
Notes   41

**3 Economic Dimensions of Health Care and
Principles in Health Policy**..**43**

Introduction   43
Why Health is of Value and Why Health Expenditures
    Should Rise   43
Household Behaviour and the Social Demand for Health   44
    Policy Influence   45
Efficient Production of Health   47
    Peculiar Aspects of Health Care   48
The Distributional Aspects of Health Policy   51
The Validity and Necessity of Benefit-Cost Analysis
    in Health Care Analysis   53
Principles in Health Policy   55

Principle One: Optimal Allocation of Resources into
Health Care 55
Principle Two: Optimal Balance between Prevention
and Treatment 56
Principle Three: Optimal Balance between Financial
Accessibility and Quality 56
Principle Four: The Least Burden Principle 58
Principle Five: Discount for the Poor Principle 59
Conclusions 59
Notes 59

4 The Available Policy Options 61

Introduction 61
The Moral Hazard Problem (Consumer Side) 62
General Discussion 62
Policy Options 62
The Moral Hazard Problem (Producer Side) 65
General Discussion 65
Policy Options 65
The Human Capital Investment Problem 69
Risk Management 70
General Discussion 70
Policy Options 71
Choice and Autonomy 73
General Discussion 73
Policy Options 75
Total Burden and How it is Shared 77
General Discussion 77
Policy Options 78
Conclusions 80
Notes 81

5 Recommendations 83

Introduction 83
A Universal Excess Burden Health Insurance Plan (UEBHIP) 84
Universal Insurance for All 84
User Charges 85
Choice for Better Services 87
Administrative Problems 88
Better Quality than Currently Possible 89
Private Health Insurance 89

The Role of Private Health Care Providers 90
   Tax-paid Doctors as Patient Advocates 91
Cost Containment, Global Budget Caps, and
   Malpractice Compensation 92
Autonomy and Freedom of Choice 94
Conclusions 96
Notes 97

6 Epilogue **99**
Alternative Viable Models: the Singapore Model
   and Hay's Model 99
The Workability of UEBHIP 101
Advertising and the Future of the Health Care Market 102
A Medical Ombudsman for Hong Kong? 103
Conclusions 104

Foreword

The key to the economic success of Hong Kong has been a business and policy environment which is simple, predictable and transparent. Experience shows that prosperity results from policies that protect private property rights, maintain open and competitive markets, and limit the role of the government.

The rapid structural change of Hong Kong's economy in recent years has generated considerable debate over the proper role of economic policy in the future. The restoration of sovereignty over Hong Kong from Britain to China has further complicated the debate. Anxiety persists as to whether the pre-1997 business and policy environment of Hong Kong will continue.

During this period of economic and political transition in Hong Kong, various interested parties will be re-assessing Hong Kong's existing economic policies. Inevitably, they will advocate an agenda aimed at altering the present policy making framework to reshape the future course of public policy.

For this reason, it is of paramount importance for those familiar with economic affairs to reiterate the reasons behind the success of the economic system in the past, to identify what the challenges are for the future, to analyze and understand the economy sector by sector, and to develop appropriate policy solutions to achieve continued prosperity.

In a conversation with my colleague Y. F. Luk, we came upon the idea of inviting economists from universities in Hong Kong to take up the challenge of examining systematically the economic policy issues of Hong Kong. An expanding group of economists (The Hong Kong Economic Policy Studies Forum) met several times to give form and shape to our initial ideas. The Hong Kong Economic Policy Studies Project was then launched in 1996 with some 30 economists from the universities in Hong Kong and a few from overseas. This is the first time in Hong Kong history that a concerted public effort has been undertaken by academic economists in the territory. It represents a joint expression of our collective concerns, our hopes for a better Hong Kong, and our faith in the economic future.

The Hong Kong Centre for Economic Research is privileged to be co-ordinating this Project. The unfailing support of many distinguished citizens in our endeavour and their words of encouragement are especially gratifying. We also thank the directors and editors of the City University of Hong Kong Press and The Commercial Press (H.K.) Ltd. for their enthusiasm and dedication which extends far beyond the call of duty.

Yue-Chim Richard Wong
Director
The Hong Kong Centre
for Economic Research

Foreword by the Series Editor

Judging from the end results, health care services in Hong Kong can be taken as quite satisfactory. The health conditions of Hong Kong citizens compare favourably with those in advanced economies, and life expectancies of both males and females in Hong Kong rank among the top in the world. Yet, to come up with these accomplishments, Hong Kong people have put in vast amounts of resources in health care. It is thus natural to ask whether the resources put into health care are efficiently allocated, and whether health care services can be further improved given the current input of resources.

On the demand side, population in Hong Kong have been growing fast recently relative to the past, and they have also been ageing constantly. These have greatly increased the demand for health care. At the same time, new medical techniques and discoveries have raised the likelihood of curing some previously fatal diseases. However, health care services are by no means homogeneous in nature. Treatments of chronic illnesses suffered by the elderly and new medical techniques and equipment are in general very expensive. Health care services in Hong Kong have to face the challenge of increasing demand at increasing costs.

Most Hong Kong people turn to the public clinics and hospitals for health care. Hong Kong's public health care system is huge and accounts for a great share of government budget every year. Will the government have to keep funding increasing expenditures in health care, and how would this be financed? Should it raise tax revenues, or should other social services be curtailed? Should the general public shoulder their own spending, or should they be encouraged to rely more on health care insurance? Can there be better co-ordination between the public and private health care systems for more efficient resource allocation?

This book is the result of research and analysis of the above issues and queries. The author, Professor Lok Sang Ho, explores how resources in health care can be better utilized without lowering the standard of services. He also proposes an innovative financing scheme to handle the expected, ever increasing, health-care expenditures. His discussion is based on economic analysis as well as results from a large survey of households, medical doctors, and hospital administrators.

Professor Ho's proposal of financing health care strikes a balance between money from the public purse and money from the consumers' own pockets, while at the same time allowing the consumers the flexibility to choose the level of health care they find desirable and affordable. Health care services are important for the physical well being of the people, but they also account for a large proportion of economic resources. Professor Ho's analysis and proposal are worthy of attention by policy-makers and the concerned public.

Y. F. Luk
School of Economics and Finance
The University of Hong Kong

Preface

Financial support from the Hong Kong Centre of Economic Research is gratefully acknowledged. The author wants to thank Dr. Fung Hong, Miss Nancy Tse, Mr. Geoffrey Lieu, and Miss Anita Mau, all of the H.K. Hospital Authority, for their assistance in the present study. Special words of thanks are extended to the doctors and Hospital Chief Executives of the Hospital Authority who responded in our surveys, and the same words are extended to those doctors and hospital administrators from the private sector who so kindly responded.

Thanks are also due to Dr. Li Pang Kwong of the Survey Research Programme of Lingnan College, who provided technical help and to Professor Ake Blomqvist and Professor William Liu who gave valuable suggestions. The author also wishes to thank all staff of the Centre for Public Policy Studies for their assistance throughout the project. At the planning stage of the Project, I gained insights from discussions with Professor S.H. Lee of The Chinese University of Hong Kong.

Last but not least, I want to thank my friend, Dr. Vansen Lee, who gave me some ideas at one time, and Dr. Paul Kwong of the City University Press for editorial suggestions.

Lok Sang Ho
Professor and Director
Centre for Public Policy Studies
Lingnan College

List of Illustrations

Figures

Figure 1.1   Growth of Resource Input, 1986–95   13

Figure 1.2   General vs Specialist Outpatients   14

Figure 1.3   Bed Adequacy vs Bed Occupancy   14

Tables

Table 1.1   Death Rates in 10 Major Hospital Authority   4
             Hospitals, 1994–96

Table 1.2   Ageing and Demographic Trends in Hong Kong,   5
             1986–2016

Table 1.3   Average Working Hours for Doctors   6

Table 1.4   Perception of Impact of Resource Constraint,   6
             Doctors in Public vs Private Hospitals

Table 1.5a   Health Care Expenditures Relative to GDP, Hong   8
             Kong vs Other Countries

Table 1.5b   Public Expenditures on Health Care Spending as %   10
             of GDP

Table 1.6   Hospitalization Rates, Hong Kong, 1989–95   11

Table 1.7a   Utilization Rates and Resource Input, 1986–95   12

Table 1.7b   Status of Hospital Bed Supply & Activities,   16
             Hospital Authority, 1995–97

Table 2.1   Recurrent Budget of Hospital Authority, 1996–97   121

Table 2.2a   Market Share in Terms of Inpatients, 1985–95   122

Table 2.2b   Market Share in Terms of Inpatient Days, 1985–96   122

Table 2.3a   Overall Satisfaction Indicators, Public vs Private 123
             Hospitals

Table 2.3b   Overall Satisfaction Indicators, Frequency of   123
             Expression of Satisfaction

Table 2.4a	Quality of Care as Perceived by Hospital Authority Doctors	124
Table 2.4b	Quality of Care as Perceived by Private Hospital Doctors	124
Table 2.5	Those Preferring Private Hospital by Household Income	125
Table 2.6	Willingness to Pay More Taxes to Get Better Services	125
Table 2.7	Those Willing to Pay More Taxes for Better Services by Household Income Categories	126
Table 2.8	Those Willing to Pay More Taxes for Better Services by Age Distribution	126
Table 2.9	Public Hospital Fees, 1995 and 1996	127
Table 2.10	In-patients by Charges Paid and by Type of Hospital, 1991	127
Table 2.11	Degree of Financial Difficulty in Meeting Medical Expenses	128
Table 2.12	Percentage of Households Potentially at Financial Risk	128
Table 2.13	Regression of "Not Worried Index" against Age & Income	129
Table 2.14	Domestic Households by Monthly Household Income, 1986, 1991, 1996	129
Table 2.15a	Median Charges for Private Practitioners, 1996	130
Table 2.15b	Actual Charges for one Private Hospital Patient, November 1996	131
Table 2.16a	Doctor's Ratings of Professional Autonomy in Hong Kong's Hospitals	132
Table 2.16b	Professional Autonomy in Hong Kong's Hospitals	132
Table 2.17	Reasons Cited for Preference by Frequency Cited	133
Table 2.18	Attrition Rates for Workers in HA, 1995 and 1996	133
Table 3.1	Decline in Job-related Health Insurance Coverage in the U.S., 1970 and 1992	51
Table 4.1	Premiums of Blue Cross Medical Insurance	73
Table 5.1	Yearly Health Spending Limits for a Typical Hong Kong Household	86

Table 6.1   Impact of the Medisave Plan of Singapore, 1982–94   100
Table 6.2   Fees of Primary Care Services Supplied by   104
             Department of Health, HA Hospitals

CHAPTER 1

Introduction

"Take my state, Colorado. . . Over 50 percent of our hospital beds are empty; we have twenty-one hospitals doing open heart surgery, and three doing transplants (three times what is needed). We have (for 3.5 million people) more MRI machines than Canada, and far too many specialists. This [happens] in a state in which 450,000 citizens are uninsured and another 400,000 citizens underinsured. We have a large excess capacity in neonatology, yet 21 percent of our women give birth without adequate prenatal care. Excess capacity sits cheek-by-jowl with great need."

> Richard D. Lamm,
> Director, Center for Public
> Policy & Contemporary Issues,
> University of Denver, State of
> Colorado, USA.[1]

The sorry state of health affairs of Colorado in 1994, and that of many American States today, are not an uncommon phenomenon. Even in China, a country that is grossly under-provided with health care services, pockets of urban areas can be found in which expensive medical equipment are under-utilized. Closer at home in Hong Kong, private sector hospitals are generally flush with excess capacity too. The average utilization rate of beds in private hospitals was 34.3%, much lower than the 81.24% average reported for Hospital Authority (HA) hospitals, according to the results of our survey of 14 hospitals. Granted that the number of private hospitals surveyed by us is small (only three), our conclusion about the excess capacity of private hospitals was nevertheless sound and significant because this conclusion is supported indirectly by the fact that 12 private hospitals had signed a joint petition to urge the government to cut back its subsidies to the more affluent patients of the government's Hospital Authority (HA) so that private hospitals could survive (see Editorial, *Ming Pao*, 7 June 1996).[2]

One important task of health care reform in Hong Kong is clearly to provide a framework for optimal interfacing between the private and public health care sectors, and to improve the efficiency of utilizing existing resources within the private and public sectors. In search of such a feasible framework, we have analyzed the past and present developments in Chapter 2 and presented several options for future policy development in Chapters 4 through 5. At this point, it would be instructive to review the roots of the current crises facing the Hospital Authority (HA) and the health system.

The interfacing of the private and public sectors in health care was very much the focus of attention in the *Scott Report* (1985), which was a comprehensive review, commissioned by the Hong Kong government, of the medical care sector. The *Scott Report* provided the groundwork for the establishment of the present Hospital Authority. The report's main recommendation was that the government hospitals and subvented hospitals should be separated from the Hospital Services Department and they should be managed by a nonprofit-making, statutory body (the Hospital Authority) set up for the purpose. It recommended the establishment of higher priced, private and semi-private wards to meet the needs of higher income people. It also suggested that government doctors be given some flexibility for outside practice operating from publicly funded facilities. Most of the recommendations of the *Scott Report* were reaffirmed in a subsequent report, the *Report of the Provisional Hospital Authority* (1989).

Hay (1992) was not optimistic that the formation of the Hospital Authority would improve substantially the quality of health care and the choice of patients. The main reason for his pessimism, quite apart from the fact that the Hospital Authority does not deal squarely with the delivery of primary care, is that the Hospital Authority still maintains a top-down, bureaucratic, command structure rather than a market-based system that is based on the motivations of private individuals. He believes that the long-term solution to the health care problem lies in the revitalization of the private sector health-care industry. His assessment seems partially correct. Already, there are visible cracks in the current system reflected in the spade of bad press about the HA.

The year 1996 was not a good year for the Hospital Authority. There were reports about mismatching of blood types during transfusions, misplacing of patient files, delayed treatment of an otherwise curable disease (malaria) leading to death, complaints of a high incidence of suffocation of newborns on delivery leading to brain damage or death, a case of multiple cancellations of scheduled surgery leading to death, a report of a rise in waiting times at specialist clinics,[3] and higher death rates in major HA hospitals (*Ming Pao* 21 June 1996). Table 1.1 shows that the rising of death rates from 29 to 37 per thousand in just two years is indicative of the general decline of quality of HA services.

To be fair, not all of these complaints are valid. In particular, according to the Hospital Authority, the rise in the death rates recorded is in part a result of the introduction of a same-day-release care scheme, and in part a result of the higher average age of patients. Healthier patients who had been formerly admitted were now taken care of under the same-day-release programme. Since they were not included in the denominator, death rates are pushed up. This explanation, however, begs other questions. While it would imply that the average stay would be longer because the earlier short-stay patients were not admitted any more, in actual fact, the average length of stay continued to fall in the year. Indeed, together with the rise in readmission rates, this suggests a tendency for premature discharge. In any case, Dr. Yip Wai Chun, then President of the Public Doctors Association, thought the HA explanation at most told only part of the story (*Ming Pao*, 22 June 1996).

Table 1.1

Death Rates* in 10 Major Hospital Authority Hospitals, 1994–96

Hospital	1994	1995	1996*
Caritas	41.29	41.67	52.66
Yan Chai	28.28	32.06	43.04
Queen Elizabeth	34.84	34.73	41.27
United	25.86	31.02	37.38
Kwong Wah	24.11	28.68	34.98
Eastern Youde	25.13	28.42	36.64
Tuen Mun	27.72	27.93	31.50
Prince of Wales	27.12	31.17	33.41
Queen Mary	27.43	26.89	29.12
Princess Margaret	29.95	28.27	29.62
Mean (across hospitals)**	29.17	31.08	36.96

Source: *Ming Pao*, 21 June 1996.

Notes: * The death rate is the proportional number of deaths (among the sum of deaths and discharges), expressed in deaths per 1000; 1996 figures are provisional.
** The simple mean is an indicative though inaccurate value of the death rate of all hospitals.

There is little doubt that the HA is fighting an uphill battle in maintaining or upgrading quality. While the HA should be commended for its effort to improve services, particularly in relating to the families of patients and in improving efficiency in general, the community's demand for better quality and higher quantity of services is running ahead of resources. The overall health care budget allocated for the fiscal year 1996–97 actually *fell* in real terms by 5.1%, even though real recurrent expenditure budget rose by 4.4%. The HA has committed a 2.5% productivity increase for the year, meaning that all service delivery units are expected to provide the same level of service with only 97.5% of the baseline budget (which allows for inflation), the savings being assigned for new service initiatives.[4] This is certainly an honourable commitment, but to expect continuous productivity improvement in a labour-intensive environment is quite unrealistic. It must be remembered that some 82% of the HA's annual budget comprises personal emoluments and staff costs. In the longer term, the prospect will be even more challenging as the population of Hong Kong grows older.

Table 1.2

Ageing and Demographic Trends in Hong Kong, 1986–2016

Year	Percentage 60 and above	Percentage 65 and above	Child Dependency Ratio (1)	Elderly Dependency Ratio (2)
1986	N.A.	7.6	333	109
1991	13.0	8.7	296	124
1996	14.1	10.0	266	141
2001*	14.4	10.8	228	149
2006*	14.8	11.2	211	153
2011*	17.0	11.4	197	154
2016*	19.8	13.3	200	184

Source: *1996 Population By-census: Summary Results*, 1996 and *Hong Kong Population Projections 1997–2016*, Census and Statistics Department, 1997.

Notes: (1) The number of persons aged under 15 per 1,000 persons in the 15–64 age group. (2) The number of persons aged 65 and over per 1,000 persons in the 15–64 age group.
* 1997 projections.

Table 1.2 provides an indication of Hong Kong's demographic trends. Clearly, Hong Kong's population is ageing. According to a rule of thumb based on a range of observations for the early 1980s reported in OECD (1994), persons aged over 65 consume about four times as much health care as those below 65. The continuing ageing of the Hong Kong population is exerting tremendous pressure on the existing health care system. As this pressure mounts, *de facto* rationing of resources is inevitable. Patients will be selectively admitted and discharged and treated or denied treatment according to some benefit-cost rule that may not correspond with the wishes of either the patients or their families.[5]

A manifestation of this mounting pressure on the HA system is found in the statistics of working hours. Table 1.3 shows that roughly half of all HA doctors work an average of 60 hours or more per week. Of these, slightly less than half work over 70 hours per week. These figures are much higher than the corresponding figures for the private sector. HA doctors are known to work more intensively than private doctors, to the extent that both HA doctors

Chapter 1

Table 1.3
Average Working Hours for Doctors*

Average Working Hours per week	% among HA Doctors	% among non-HA Doctors
Below 40	0.0	4.9
40–49	32.3	42.6
50–59	16.9	18.0
60–69	26.5	19.7
70 and Over	23.8	14.8

Source: Doctors' Survey, December 1996.

Notes: *188 among 189 HA doctors surveyed reported working hours. All of the 61 non-HA doctors reported working hours. The average number of working hours in HA hospitals may be understated by a sampling bias because major hospitals, including the Queen Mary Hospital and the Queen Elizabeth Hospital, indicated that their doctors were too busy to respond to the survey. HA means Hospital Authority (public hospitals).

Table 1.4
Perception of Impact of Resource Constraint, Doctors in Public vs Private Hospitals

Statement	Percentage of "Agree" or "Very Much Agree"	Percentage of "Disagree" or "Very Much Disagree"
Workload has jeopardized the quality of care	76.9 (among HA doctors)	10.4 (among HA doctors)
	18.7 (among Non-HA doctors)	39.8 (among Non-HA doctors)
Nursing support is adequate	9.2 (among HA doctors	61.7 (among HA doctors)
	21.8 (among Non-HA doctors)	31.4 (among Non-HA doctors)
Patients are seldom denied appropriate care because of a lack of resources	49.2 (among HA doctors)	21.6 (among HA doctors)
	38.0 (among Non-HA doctors)	24.0 (among Non-HA doctors)

Source: Doctors' Survey, December 1996.

Notes: Percentages are based on valid responses; missing values excluded.

and non-HA doctors agree that the heavy workload of HA doctors is far more likely to jeopardize the quality of care than that of non-HA doctors (Table 1.4, Table 2.4 in Appendix C).

The foregoing depiction of the situation, we see that the health care system in Hong Kong is now at a crossroads. With demand outstripping supply in the public sector, the HA system is under stress. Both quality of care and quantity of care are increasingly at risk. On the other hand, idle capacity in many private hospitals implies waste and inefficiency. Should these trends continue and worsen, then quite soon the ridiculous situation in Colorado (p. 1), could be replicated in Hong Kong.

Clearly, the status quo is no longer viable. To relieve the stress within the existing system, additional resources have to be mobilized. Raising taxes to improve quality and quantity will, however, accelerate the demise of private hospitals and may encourage an unhealthy lifestyle and overconsumption of publicly financed health care services. In any case, the tax increases required will be large and will not be allowed under the Basic Law. Increasing user charges will raise the spectre of possible financial stress for patients and their families. The idea has been opposed bitterly by the community, largely because the potential burden could be difficult to absorb for some households. What else then, is to be done?

This book looks at the key issue of how to raise the resources needed to meet the expectations of the public and the increasing demands due to the phenomena of ageing and population expansion. The main questions to answer are:

1. How should the additional, needed funds be raised?
2. How should the burden be divided?
3. How should the incentive of caregivers to work efficiently in the interest of patients be preserved?
4. How should the incentive of citizens to adopt a more healthy lifestyle be preserved?
5. How much should be devoted to improving Hong Kong's health care infrastructure, to improving existing services, and to illness prevention?

Table 1.5a

Health Care Expenditures Relative to GDP, Hong Kong vs Other Countries

	1991	1992	1993	1994	1995
Public health care expenditure as % of GDP	1.67	1.75	2.06	1.91	2.16
Private health care expenditure as % of GDP	2.11	2.19	2.15	2.42	2.65
Health care expenditure as % of GDP (**Hong Kong**)	**3.78**	**3.94**	**4.21**	**4.32**	**4.81**
Health care expenditure as % of GDP (**Other Countries**)	7.4 (European Union)[a]	8.4 (OECD average)[b]	3.2 (Singapore)[c]		

Source: *Hong Kong*, official review of the year by the HK government, various years.
          National Income Section, Census and Statistics Department, (a): Abel–Smith
          and others (1995); (b): Oxley and MacFarlan (1994); (c): Kwa (1996)

Note: Public health care expenditure for 1991 refers to fiscal year 1991–1992.
          GDP figures refer to calendar year.

6. What should the roles of private sector health service providers and insurers be?

Before attempting a comparison of various alternatives to the present health system, we need to grasp the basics of the present system and to appreciate the magnitude of our current problems in terms of various rates of supply and usage. The remainder of this introductory chapter is devoted to that task. Further information about the financing of private and HA hospitals are provided in Chapter 2 in which a report on the findings of a household survey of health care opinions is also given. The survey findings, along with other evidence, are the input to an evaluative framework of the present health system. Building on the findings of Chapters 1 and 2, Chapter 3 discusses the economic dimensions of health care and the principles of health policy. Chapter 4 discusses policy options. Chapter 5 presents our recommendations. We especially recommend setting up a Universal Excess Burden Health Insurance Plan

(UEBHIP) for Hong Kong. Chapter 6 in the form of an epilogue compares the proposed system with alternative policy options and discusses.. additional reforms.

The Present System under Stress

Health care services in Hong Kong are jointly supplied by the public and the private sectors. In 1995 about 2.16% of the territory's gross domestic product was devoted to public sector health care services (see Table 1.5a). This comprises both capital and recurrent expenditures, and includes expenditures made by the Department of Health and the Hospital Authority. An estimated 2.65% of the GDP was attributable to the private sector. Total spending on health care, according to this calculation, amounted to about 4.81% of GDP.

Table 1.5a shows that health expenditures in both public and private sectors have been rising steadily — generally at a pace faster than the GDP. As recently as 1991, only 3.78% of the GDP consisted of health care. By 1995 this figure had gone up to 4.81%.

This rapid increase in health care expenditures is causing concern. In a substantive sense, however, this increase in health care expenditures may be efficient and in itself may not be a problem. As Hong Kong becomes more affluent and as its population ages, the government is expected to devote more resources to health care because that is what consumers want and need. In an affluent society, access to the latest production and consumption technology means that the cost of time lost during sickness in terms of lost production and consumption opportunities is very high. Among OECD countries, a recent estimate of the income elasticity of demand for health care is 0.74 (Oxley and MacFarlan 1994, p. 97). There are no estimates of the income elasticity of demand for Hong Kong, but as Hong Kong has achieved today's affluence in a relatively short time and as health services had been under-supplied, there is catching up to do.

With the notable exception of Singapore, Hong Kong's health care spending, if the official statistics can be believed, is very low

Table 1.5b
Public Expenditures on Health Care Spending as % of GDP

Country / Region	1986	1989	1991	1992	1993	1994	1995
Hong Kong	**1.38**	**1.39**	**1.67**	**1.75**	**2.06**	**1.91**	**2.16**
European Union			5.79				
Singapore	1.00	0.90					
United Kingdom				5.99			

Source: *Hong Kong*, various issues.
         Singapore data from *Yearbook of Statistics*, cited in Phua Kai Hong:
         Privatization and Restructuring of Health Services in Singapore.
         European Union data based on OECD data cited in Table 2.2 in Abel–Smith,
         Figueras, Holland, McKee, and Mossialos (1995).
Note: The figures for Hong Kong health care expenditures in the public sector for
         a year refer to fiscal year starting in that year; GDP figures are for the
         calendar year.

relative to the GDP by international standards. As Hay pointed out, some cost items were omitted. Official figures on public health care expenditures grossly underestimate resource consumption because the imputed rental value of buildings and facilities has not been included; at the same time the value of services supplied gratis by other government departments has been either not fully reflected or not accounted for at all (Hay 1992, p. 10).

The efficiency of Hong Kong's health care system is apparent from the most frequently used indicators of health (such as life expectancy and infant mortality rate), notwithstanding the tiny percentage of public health care spending in the gross domestic product. Admittedly, as was also pointed out by Hay (1992), health indicators depend as much on lifestyle as on public expenditure, and Hong Kong's public spending on health care is grossly understated. Still, even doubling the official figures is unlikely to take Hong Kong away from the ranks of countries with relatively low spending on health care.

Table 1.6
Hospitalization Rates, Hong Kong, 1989–95

Age Group	Oct.–Dec. 89	July–Sept. 91	April–Aug. 95	Increase since 1989 (%)
0– 4	27.7	35.4	50.7	+83.0
5–14	7.7	8.3	12.0	+55.8
15–24	11.2	10.7	13.7	+22.3
25–34	24.2	27.3	28.8	+19.0
35–44	17.2	17.5	28.5	+65.7
45–54	18.6	18.8	31.6	+69.9
55–64	28.0	29.9	38.9	+38.9
65+	50.7	47.3	66.7*	+31.5
Overall	20.8	22.0	30.4	+46.2

Source: Census and Statistics Department: *Report on Hospitalization Surveys*, July 1996.

Note: The rate of hospitalization per 1,000 persons is based on admittance to hospital during the six months before enumeration.
* = 2.4 times the arithmetic average of the admission rates for the 15 to 64 age group.

Table 1.5b throws some light on the efficiency issue. Caution must be exercised, however, in making cross-country comparisons. Accounting methods may differ, and a relatively younger population may also explain in part the lower spending on health care for some countries. Compared to most industrial nations, Hong Kong's population is considered young.[6]

Over the years, hospitalization rates for all age groups within the population of Hong Kong have increased (Table 1.6). In principle this can be a result of either a rise in the incidence of hospital admissions across the population or a rise in the incidence of multiple admissions. The former may be a result of rising expectations or knowledge about the need for admissions, higher availability of hospital beds, or a general deterioration of health conditions. The latter may be a result of patients requiring more admissions, which in turn could be a result of premature discharge of patients or a deterioration in the health conditions of patients. It seems unlikely that health conditions across the population or those

Table 1.7a
Utilization Rates and Resource Input, 1986–95

Resource Input	1986	1989	1991	1992	1993	1994	1995
1 Doctors per capita	0.93	1.06	1.14	1.18	1.21	1.27	1.32
2 Beds (incl. private) per capita	4.4	4.4	4.4	4.5	4.5	4.6	4.7
3 Registered nurses, public sector (general) per capita	1.05	1.12	1.63	1.65	1.71	1.76	1.80
4 Registered nurses, private, (general) per capita	1.71	2.05	1.86	1.95	2.00	2.06	2.09
5 Enrolled general nurses, public sector per capita	0.24	0.24	0.45	0.47	0.48	0.50	0.52
6 Enrolled general nurses, private sector per capita	0.74	0.88	0.77	0.82	0.86	0.88	0.89
Utilization Rates							
7 Bed adequacy ratio (beds per 1000 / hospitalization rate*)		0.21	0.20				0.15
8 General outpatient attendance (DH) / population	1.00	0.98	0.95	0.94	0.93	0.90	0.91
9 Special outpatient attendance (HA) / population	0.47	0.49	0.51	0.53	0.57	0.61	0.66
10 Inpatient bed occupancy rate (HA)					79.6	80.6	81.8**

Source: *Hong Kong Annual Digest of Statistics* 1996. Also Department of Health (DH), and Hospital Authority (HA).

Notes: * Based on hospitalization rates published in *Report on Hospitalization Surveys*, Statistics and Information Section, Hospital Authority Head Office, July 1996. **In-patient bed occupancy rate based on *HK Monthly Digest of Statistics*. Number of nurses in the private sector may include inactive nurses.

of hospitalized patients have on average worsened over the years. The possibility cannot be ruled out that some patients are being discharged prematurely on account of resource considerations.

Table 1.6 gives us a glimpse of the effect of ageing on health care costs. According to the table, the hospitalization rate for the 65+ group was much higher than that of any other age group. For 1995, for example, at 66.7 per 1000, the hospitalization rate was 2.34 times the rate for the 25–34 group and over five times the hospitalization rate for the 5–14 group.

Figure 1.1
Growth of Resource Input, 1986–95

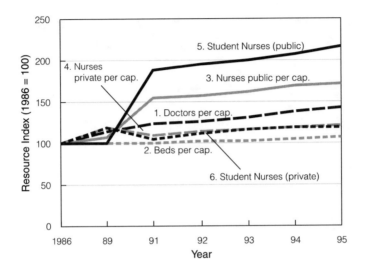

Although the government has allocated more and more public money to health care (from 1.39% of GDP in 1989 to 2.16% of GDP in 1995), Hong Kong's health care facilities and health care professionals are actually facing unprecedented pressure to meet rising demands.

Rows 1 to 6 in Table 1.7a show that the resource-to-population ratios appear to show steady improvement in recent years.(Figure 1.1) Notwithstanding an increase in the number of doctors, beds, and nurses relative to the population, the rate of utilization of the available resources has increased sharply. Row 7 shows the ratio of the beds per thousand population to the hospitalization rate. This ratio has declined noticeably since 1990. The inpatient bed occupancy rate is rising while the number of clinical attendance per capita is rising rapidly both for general clinic attendance and for specialist clinic attendance (Figures 1.2 to 1.3).

Against this background, internal targets within the Hospital Authority to reduce waiting times for first appointments at 90% of specialist clinics for consultation at specialist clinics, for major elective surgery, and for cataract surgery, failed to be met as of 31

Figure 1.2
General vs Specialist Outpatients

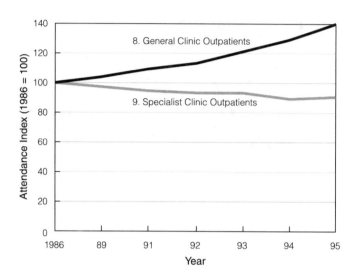

Figure 1.3
Bed Adequacy vs Bed Occupancy

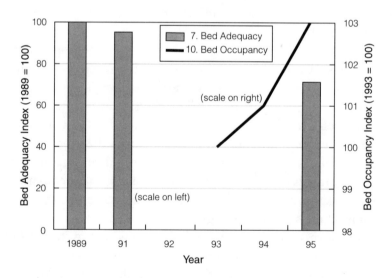

Source:　　Table 1.7a for Figure 1.1(row 1 to 6), 1.2 (row 8 and 9), 1.3 (row 7 and 10).

March 1995. The outlook is not at all optimistic given the continuing demographic trends of the population and the constraint of resource availability projected. Table 1.7b on the status of hospital bed supply and projected activities is based on estimates by the Hospital Authority in February 1996. It shows that in spite of a continual increase in resource commitment, the system is under increasing stress.

There is little doubt that the low cost of publicly provided medical care is one reason that the rate of utilization of health care facilities is so much higher in Hong Kong than elsewhere. This is particularly true with respect to emergency and accident department facilities, which are free. However, admission to public hospitals is subject to a *gate-keeper system,* so all public hospital admissions are based on professional judgement and cannot be attributed to consumer response to low prices. There is no reason to doubt the professional opinion of HA doctors who decide to admit patients. They have no financial gain by admitting patients, though admitting more patients will increase their workload.

With the manpower of the HA under heavy pressure over extended periods, the incidence of human error is likely to rise, and queues and covert rationing has become more prevalent. The general consensus today is that either more resources are put into medical care, or the consequence will be a decline in the quality of medical care. Although it is held widely that it is the responsibility of the government to protect the health of citizens, it is not generally appreciated that the resources available to the government must either be derived from taxpayers or be garnered by cutting back other services in order to make way for the additional medical expenditures. Yet, in the final analysis, how shall these additional resources be made available?

As a way to summarize the issues raised thus far, it is worth restating some specific questions posed in the opening of this chapter. Should more or higher taxes be imposed? Should a mandatory, universal health insurance scheme be introduced and revenue raised

Table 1.7b

Status of Hospital Bed Supply & Activities, Hospital Authority, 1995–97

Bed Supply	As at March 31 1995 (Actual)	As at March 31 1996 (Estimate)	As at March 31 1997 (Plan)
Total number of hospital beds	24,166	25,117	25,974
general	17,240	17,677	18,250
infirmary	1,462	1,772	1,927
mentally ill	4,639	4,843	4,945
mentally handicapped	825	825	825
Number of psychiatric day places	575	575	615
Number of geriatric day places	325	415	455

Hospital Bed Activities	1994–95 (Actual)	1995–96 (Estimate)	1996–97 (Estimate)
Total attendance at accident & emergency departments	1,733,040	1,912,300	1,985,400
General in–patient services			
Number of in–patients discharged	832,281	900,600	989,100
Average bed occupancy rate (%)	79.2	81.4	82.8
Average length of stay (days)	7.8	7.7	7.3
Mentally–ill inpatient services			
Number of in–patients discharged	1,556,234	1,586,700	1,646,800
Average bed occupancy rate (%)	94.6	91.1	91.1
Average length of stay (days)	193.7	184.2	183.2
Mentally–handicapped inpatient services			
Number of in–patients discharged	234,588	257,300	259,800
Average bed occupancy rate (%)	78.1	83.4	84.4
Average length of stay (days)	531.9	89.9	575.9
Outpatient attendance			
Specialist outpatient clinics	5,139,710	5,538,600	6,005,500
General outpatient clinics	741,298	732,100	713,800
Community services (home visits and attendance)			
Community nurse visits	289,224	330,900	347,300
Psychiatric day centre	100,869	109,500	113,400
Geriatric day centre	62,653	75,600	84,000

Source: *Budget Allocation 1996 / 97*, Hospital Authority: Finance Committee, endorsed on 29 February 1996.

through insurance premiums? Should patient fees be raised? Should itemized charges be extended to more categories of expenditures? Should the poor be exempt from charges? Should other government services be cut back and taxes not raised? These questions will be addressed toward the latter part of the book where various options of reform will be considered. To anticipate somewhat, we shall argue the case for a special form of *non-contributory* health insurance.

Conclusions

Even though Hong Kong has devoted an increasing proportion of public money to health care, there will still be an imperative to increase spending on health care in order to provide for the greater needs of an ageing population and to meet the rising expectations of an increasingly affluent society. The figures suggest that the pace at which the government is increasing public spending on health care is not keeping up with the rising demands. As a result, the quality and quantity of health care provided to date appear to lag behind requirements.

Yet the health care conundrum is not to be solved simply by allocating more public money into health care. Indeed, there is no presumption that tax financing is the best way to raise the resources needed to boost quality and quantity. The principle of least burden (See Chapter 3) suggests that alternative ways of financing health care should be considered along with tax financing. Moreover, there has to be a mechanism that ensures that the money spent on health care is spent in the right amount in the right area. This task cannot be taken up by bureaucrats alone, but rather must rely on the judgement of medical professionals operating in an environment that gives them the incentive to do so.

Notes

1. Hastings Center Report, November / December 1994, p. 14.

2. Baptist Hospital later withdrew from the list of signatories.

3. According to the report, the waiting times for specialist outpatient appointments had gone up during the year 1995–96: from 4 weeks to 7.5 weeks for psychiatry; from 4 weeks to almost 7 weeks for paediatrics; from 6 weeks to almost 9 weeks for gynaecology; from 14 weeks to 19 weeks for ophthalmology; from 6.5 weeks to 11 weeks for orthopedics; and from 7 weeks to 9 weeks for surgery.

4. See *Budget Allocation 1996 / 97*, Finance Committee of the Hospital Authority for endorsement on 29 February 1996.

5. In principle there is nothing wrong with applying a benefit-cost rule. However, when resources are constrained, the cost of treating a patient is not the cost of the resources — which the patient and his family may be willing to shoulder. The cost becomes the treatment of another patient. If this other patient has a better chance to survive for a longer period as a result of the treatment, doctors may decide to treat him (her) rather than the first patient.

6. According to Hay (1992), the median age of the population in Hong Kong was 28. It was 32.3 which "had a 50% greater proportion of people over 65 than Hong Kong."(p. 2, p. 14).

CHAPTER 2

The Current Health Care System

Introduction

According to a recent study by the Census and Statistics Department (See *Monthly Digest of Statistics*, May 1996), 90% of patients admitted to public hospitals do not have any health insurance coverage. It is precisely because they have been effectively and publicly insured under the present health care system that they have little need to seek private insurance. In 1996 patients were responsible for only 3.17% of total recurrent costs in Hong Kong's public hospitals. So in a substantive sense it can be said that the hospitalization costs of Hong Kong people who choose public hospitals in case of need are underwritten by the taxpayers. The insurance premiums are effectively paid by *themselves* to the extent that they pay more taxes than otherwise, thus effectively incorporating the insurance premium. These premiums are effectively paid by *others* for those whose tax burden has not been increased by virtue of the health care system. Such people are sheltered from the burden of the insurance premium by virtue of distributive considerations.

In a substantive sense, this insurance system operates like a giant Health Maintenance Organization (HMO). In Hong Kong, the Hospital Authority (HA) runs a system of some 40 hospitals with a total of well over 24,000 hospital beds. It is funded by taxpayers through a "capitation mechanism" to look after their hospitalization needs. Capitation is a prepayment system whereby an HMO gets the funds expected to be needed in order to look after the health of enrollees. The Hospital Authority in 1996–97 had a budget of HK$20,001 million inclusive of income arising from charges and donations. Exclusive of the latter, direct budget allocation from the government amounted to $19,225 million (see Table 2.1*). This system contrasts with the fee-for-service arrangement whereby patients are expected to come up with the funds needed when they are hospitalized. The distinguishing feature of an HMO is that it is simultaneously the insurer and the service provider. The HA, in a substantive sense then, is a giant HMO, but one that is not profit-making. The government is a middleman effectively enrolling all Hong Kong residents into the HMO and transferring enrollment fees to the HA.

Since all Hong Kong residents with a valid Hong Kong identity card are eligible for the subsidized services of the HA, and since all Hong Kong residents are subject to tax, the "giant HMO" in Hong Kong is clearly not based on voluntary participation and enrollment. Universal coverage means that those who are known to suffer from chronic health problems will not be excluded from service. Exclusion of certain people generally characterizes unregulated HMOs in a free market.[1] Because of much lower cost relative to the private hospital system and universal access to care in the public hospital system, about 84% of patients opted for public hospitals (Table 2.2a).[2] Nevertheless, private hospitals are still considered the better choice for most patients if cost is not the consideration.[3]

The funding of the HA, as well as that of government-operated primary care clinics, is derived exclusively from taxes. The public health system of Hong Kong unavoidably puts great pressure on the government to increase taxes, given the expected increase in costs stemming from: (1) the ageing of the population, (2) the availability of advanced but expensive technology and drugs, and (3) the rising expectations of the community. Yet, as Hong Kong is committed to low taxes under the Basic Law, the HA is forced to look for alternative sources of funds, to ration services, or else to compromise the quality of services provided.

---

* All tables in Chapter 2 are given in the Appendix C starting on page 121 .

A caveat should be added, which is that the possibility for efficiency or productivity improvement exists. Such an improvement allows the opportunity trade-off line between quality and quantity to move out (implying an improvement in quality and/or quantity) without necessarily involving an increase in burden. As far as policy is concerned, however, we should adopt a principle of rewarding improvements in efficiency and maintaining incentives to further improve efficiency, rather than demoralizing staff by imposing excessive, increasingly onerous demands to raise productivity.

The Evaluative Framework

The Perennial Trade-off between Quality, Financial Accessibility, and Least Burden

Whether one likes it or not, hard choices must be faced in public policy. Unfortunately, this is not necessarily apparent to some commentators on health issues who point to the large fiscal reserves of the government in arguing that the government is devoting far too little resources to health care.

The post-1997 government no doubt has a combined fiscal reserve that is the envy of governments everywhere. The Land Fund had accumulated over HK\$150 billion to add to the fiscal reserve of close to HK\$150 billion at the time Hong Kong SAR Government was formed on 1 July 1997. However, the government is the custodian of the interest not only of this generation but that of future generations. The government must also balance the needs of health care against the needs of education, social welfare, public security, infrastructure development, housing, and so on. Rising recurrent expenditures that are not financed by recurrent income will finally eat up any fiscal reserve, impairing the government's ability to withstand crises as well as fluctuations in business confidence.

In principle, one goal must be the optimal allocation of resources to health care. This means resources should be allocated to health care as long as they produce more benefit than that arising from alternative uses, such as housing and education. The value of the alternative uses forgone, or the opportunity cost of resources allocated to health care, represents the total burden placed on the entire society.

In general, if people are willing to accept the increase in burden involved, it is possible, by increasing the resources allocated to health care, to improve both the quality of health care and the quantity of health care services. Without increasing the amount of resources allocated to health care, quality can be improved only at the expense of quantity, and similarly quantity only at the expense of quality. Interpreting quality as the amount of health care services received by one person, and quantity as the extension of the services to more people, which would correspond to financial accessibility, it is clear that the objectives of quality, financial accessibility, and least burden are perennially in conflict with one another. The operational meaning of these objectives is set forth in the next section within an evaluative framework of health care system.

A health care system can be assessed using four criteria. These include the three criteria discussed in the last paragraph, namely, *quality of services, financial accessibility* (as opposed to physical accessibility, which is an aspect of quality) and *burden*. In addition, a new criterion will be introduced: *autonomy and freedom of choice*. Quite independently of the three-way trade-off between quality, accessibility (quantity), and the burden, a health care system may be more or less satisfactory in terms of the autonomy and freedom of choice that the system offers members of the society. A system that provides more autonomy and free choice to members of the society, both collectively and individually and other things being equal, is superior to a system that provides less autonomy and choice.[4]

The need to introduce the additional criterion of autonomy and free choice is grounded in one famous principle in economics: the Pareto Principle, which says that the improvement in the welfare of at least one person without reducing the welfare of another other person should be construed as an improvement. Allowing individuals to opt for a higher quality of health care services and to pay fully for the extra cost, hence imposing no burden on others, is therefore an improvement. Moreover, a system that gives members of society better information about the trade-off between quality, financial accessibility, and burden, so that they can make a more intelligent collective choice, is superior to a system that obscures the trade-off, that somehow prevents intelligent collective choice, or that makes a collective decision by default.

In short, to evaluate Hong Kong's health care system, it is necessary to have quality-of-service indicators, financial accessibility indicators, burden indicators, and finally, indicators to reflect the degree of autonomy and free choice that the system offers Hong Kong's citizens.

Quality of Service

The quality-of-service indicators are multidimensional and should include the following nonexhaustive list:

Accessibility indicators

1. *physical accessibility* of each kind of medical and health services; to measure this it is necessary to have an indicator of the geographic distribution of hospitals and clinics relative to the geographic distribution of population;
2. *waiting time for diagnostic services, and waiting time for treatment,* medicinal, surgical, or therapeutic, in nonemergency cases or in emergency cases.

Accuracy indicators

1. the *rate of correct diagnosis* about the nature of an ailment;
2. the *ability to make accurate diagnosis,* in the sense of being able to assess accurately the seriousness and the precise advance of a disease or injury;
3. the *degree of appropriateness of treatment,* given a correct diagnosis.

Quality of environment indicators

1. the *risks of infection for a patient* receiving diagnostic or treatment services;
2. the *environmental quality of the hospital beds and the out-patient clinics which is certainly related to the preceding dimension of quality.*

Quality of incidental service indicators

1. the *quality of follow-up services for patients discharged* from hospitals;
2. the degree of *effectiveness of communication with family;*
3. the *quality of support for family.*

Quality of management indicators

the *quality of management* throughout the health care system to ensure accountability, effective and secure record keeping, and effective linkage and communication between health care providers with different specializations, medical technologists, and other professionals; and finally,

Quality of ambulatory service indicators

1. the *speed and availability of ambulatory services* when needed;
2. the *extent to which the services provided meet the immediate needs of the patient.*

Resource and time constraint did nor permit a complete evaluation of Hong Kong's medical care system against all of these criteria. However, a public survey done on the subject in November 1996 should shed light on these criteria when they are operationalized in real life terms. A total of 907 households were successfully contacted and canvassed via the telephone for the survey, representing a success rate of 29.6%. The survey was conducted by the Survey and Research Programme of Lingnan College. The questionnaire is given in Appendix A of this book.

The main findings are presented as follows. Table 2.3a and Table 2.3b show that the public is generally satisfied with Hong Kong's hospitals over a wide range of criteria. In terms of overall performance score (Table 2.3a), private hospitals generally appear to be superior to public hospitals — except in the category "value for money", which suggests that low cost is the main attraction of public hospitals. However, looking at the frequency of expression of satisfaction (Table 2.3b), public hospitals appear to be favoured more often than private hospitals. It scored higher with the public in terms of "trust", "environment within hospital", "nursing care", as well as overall "value for money". This public perception, for its worth, offers an explanation for the recent tendency for patients to increasingly opt for public hospitals.

The area in which public hospitals perform worst is "waiting time for surgery". Other areas in which private hospitals have a clear edge over HA hospitals include "queueing time for specialist clinic attendance" and "queueing time for diagnostic services". "Shorter queueing time" has been cited as a key reason, along with "better services", for why some households expressed a preference for private hospitals over public hospitals (22% and 43% respectively among 400 citations for a reason for such a preference). On the other hand, the predominant reason for the preference of public hospitals over private hospitals is lower cost (409 citations among 619 citations, or 66%).[5]

While the above tables indicate the perception of the public about the relative performance of HA and private hospitals, Table 2.4a and Table 2.4b provide indicators about the perception about relative performance by medical professionals. Table 2.4a represents the perception of HA doctors. It shows that HA doctors generally believe that there is a shortage of nurses in both HA and private hospitals, with the shortage being more severe in HA hospitals. The latter is probably related to the much higher utilization rate of HA beds. They generally believe that both types of hospitals provide reasonably good care. They also think that there is a slightly higher chance of patients being denied the most appropriate care in private hospitals rather than in public hospitals because of a lack of resources.

Table 2.4b represents the perception of doctors in the private sector. Interestingly, there is a high degree of agreement with the perception of HA doctors. Again there is a perception of shortage of nurses in both HA and private hospitals, with the shortage being worse in HA hospitals. They generally believe that both types of hospitals provide reasonably good care. Compared with HA doctors, private sector doctors appear to be somewhat more optimistic that patients will not be denied the most appropriate care because of a lack of resources. Although they are also concerned that excessive workload would jeopardize the quality of care in public hospitals, they appear to be somewhat less worried than HA doctors.

Table 2.5 shows that households belonging to the lower income groups generally prefer public hospitals over private hospitals, while those belonging to the higher income groups tend to prefer private hospitals to public hospitals. For the entire sample, 35.4% of respondent households indicate a preference for private hospitals should a need for hospitalization arise. This is a higher percentage than the actual proportion of patients under the care of private hospitals. According to a survey of hospitalization done by the Census and Statistics Department, 27% of inpatients stayed in private hospitals (See Special Report on Hospitalization, *Monthly Digest of Statistics,* May 1996).

In the survey conducted by the author, respondents were asked whether they were willing to pay more taxes in exchange for better medical services. Assuming that the medical care system is efficient, this provides an indication of whether the quality of medical services is at an optimal level. The results of this question are tabulated in Table 2.6, while cross-tabulations against income and age of the respondent are provided in Table 2.7 and Table 2.8.

First it is possible to observe that a clear majority among all respondents (62.9%) are prepared to pay more taxes in exchange better medical services. Among those providing a valid response — those who have indicated a positive or a negative response to the question — respondents indicating a willingness to pay more taxes in exchange for better medical services actually account for over 68% of all valid responses (62.8% of the entire sample). This corresponds with similar surveys done earlier by others, and suggests that the amount of resources allocated to health care may be less than optimal.

Second, it is possible to observe that while a majority of households in each income category is prepared to pay more taxes to get better medical service. The percentage is lowest for households in the HK$45,001 to HK$100,000 per month category (Table 2.7). This result may reflect the fact that the middle income groups are subject to the largest marginal tax rates and that they interpret "paying more taxes" more negatively than either the higher income households, who are already subject to standard tax rates, or the lower income groups, who pay no or very little taxes. The lower income groups are also known to be more frequent users of public hospitals than the middle or higher income groups, and on this account, may be more willing to pay more taxes for better services. It should be noted that because of the relatively small number of respondents in the very high income categories, the result for the over $100,000 monthly income group must be taken with great caution. It is, however, significant that 71% of households in the $15,001 to $30,000 category are willing to pay more taxes in exchange for better hospital services, given that a total of 249 households in that group responded to the question.

Third, Table 2.8 indicates that willingness to pay more taxes for better medical services seems to pervade households in all phases of the life cycle of the head of the household. The strongest demand for better health care, as expressed by a willingness to pay more taxes to obtain better hospital services, is indicated for households whose respondents (the heads of the household) are aged between 40 and 49. This is the group that is likely to have elderly parents and children to look after simultaneously.

We have thus far established that the public generally finds Hong Kong's public hospitals provide good value for money but people are unhappy with the waiting time at public-sector clinics and with the waiting time for surgery. The average "trust" score is noticeably lower for public hospitals than for private hospitals, even though the percentage of households satisfied with public hospitals is higher than that of households satisfied with private hospitals. This suggests that a minority of households may have very bad experiences with or perceptions about public hospitals, so that their negative assessment of public hospitals has pulled down the average score for trust. The survey was done in November 1996, which means that some respondents were possibly influenced by some widely publicized incidents that had occurred in the year, such as a case of delayed treatment of malaria leading to death, several cases of mismatched blood transfusions, alleged cases of suffocation of newborns during delivery, and the disappearance of patients' medical files. Finally, the survey has found that most people are willing to pay more taxes in exchange for an improved health care system; this is an indication that the present quality of health services provided is less than optimal.

Financial Accessibility: Are the Poor Denied Needed Services?

The idea that health care services should be accessible or available to all, regardless of their financial circumstances, is explicitly stated in Section 38(2) of the *Public Finance Ordinance* and reiterated again in the recent consultation document *Towards Better Health* (1993) which states:

> "In order that no Hong Kong resident is denied adequate medical treatment through lack of means, designated officers in the Department of Health, Hospital Authority and Social Welfare Department are authorized in law to waive the medical fees of those who suffer genuine financial hardship? (*Towards Better Health*, p. 8)"

There is no definition of "adequate medical treatment" in the official documents. Obviously what constitutes adequate medical treatment is subject to interpretation. Depending on the interpretation, adequate medical treatment can be quite expensive. Thus there is a need to define the level of adequate medical treatment that is financially accessible to Hong Kong residents. Since there is no basis to establish a scientific definition of adequate medical treatment, a formal mechanism for public choice is necessary. The existence of a formal process that is acceptable to the community for defining the level of adequate medical treatment is an important aspect of autonomy and freedom of choice, a subject which will be discussed in the latter part of this chapter.

Abstracting for the moment from the controversial subject of what is adequate medical treatment and whether the Hong Kong health care system effectively delivers adequate medical care, it must be acknowledged that the Hong Kong health care system is remarkable in providing financial accessibility. Table 2.9 lists the public hospital fees for Hong Kong residents. It is unlikely that a Hong Kong resident will be denied access to medical care in Hong Kong's public hospitals and government-operated clinics on financial grounds.

Table 2.10, which is based on the General Household Survey, shows that less than 2% of inpatients admitted into government or government-assisted hospitals paid HK$6,000 or more in 1991. In that year, the median monthly household income of these inpatients was HK$10,530, which translates into an annual income of HK$126,360. For 98% of patients admitted into government or government-assisted hospitals, then, the typical cost of a hospitalization was 4.7% or less of median household income. With multiple admissions, or for households with incomes falling below the median, the percentage of income spent on hospitalized care would be higher. A small minority of inpatients — 0.3% and 0.4% of the patients in government and government-assisted public hospitals respectively — spent over HK$15,000, which was about 11.87% of their mean annual household income. Unfortunately, it is not known how many of these high-cost patients were rich individuals having opted for first class or private room services and how many of them were lower income individuals having to pay for more expensive items that were subject to charges. The Director of Hospital Services at the time and the Hospital Authority of today, however, may waive the costs for the very poor. As a rule, public-assistance recipients are exempt from all charges. Overall, then, financial accessibility does not appear to be a serious problem.

Roughly 6% of all inpatients in 1991, including those in the private sector, paid HK$15,000 or more for hospitalized care. On the other hand, focusing on inpatients in private hospitals, those paying HK$15,000 or more accounted for 18.1% of all patients. Given that the median monthly income of patients in private hospitals was HK$16,615, implying an annual income of HK$199,380, it can be said that 18.1% of private hospital patients paid 7.52% or more of their median household income *on one hospitalization*. Clearly the probability of excessive burden is much higher among these patients.

Table 2.11 provides an analysis of those who reported having difficulty meeting health care expenses. For the sample of 907 responding households, 58 (6.4%) reported having had difficulty financing medical care within the past two years. Out of the 58 households, 34 reported having borrowed money to meet health care expenses. Of those who reported having difficulty meeting health care expenses, the majority reported spending 9% or more of their income on health care.

In the survey, an attempt was made to gauge the percentage of household income that can be spent on health care without significantly affecting the quality of life of households. A total of 487 respondents out of the full sample of 907 answered the question. Table 2.12 shows the percentages of households potentially at financial risk when different percentages of income are spent on health care. The table suggests that if the percentage of spending on health care accounts for 6% or less of income, 24.6% would be potentially at risk. There is a big jump of the percentage of households potentially at risk if spending on health care increases from 9% to 10% — a result apparently related to a "rounding" problem in reporting. Certainly Table 2.12 does not pretend to give a definitive answer to the question of what amount of health care spending is "affordable". It does suggest, however, that a maximum of 6% of household income being spent on health care would probably be acceptable to the majority of households in Hong Kong.

It may be thought that patients in private hospitals have the option to seek services in public hospitals, and that the fact that they voluntarily opt for private hospitals means that they can afford it. This interpretation, unfortunately, may not be correct if hospital services in the public sector are effectively rationed. With the exception of life-threatening or immediate emergencies, patients generally have to wait longer for surgery in a public hospital. The prospect of having to use the services of a much more expensive private hospital in case the queue for public hospital services is too long is certainly one reason behind the sizeable percentage (33.3%) of householders sampled in our survey indicating being worried or very much worried about unforeseen medical expenses. When including those indicating they are "somewhat worried", the ratio rises to 54.8% among all responding households. As Table 2.13 indicates, householders who are the youngest and those who have the highest income tend to be the least worried. To put it another way, this means that lower income households and especially those whose heads are older are most worried. A statistical analysis of the data shows that sex of the respondent does not affect the "not worried index".

Another consideration of the performance of a health system is concerned with the length of stay in hospitals. Admitted patients may be discharged sooner than is in their best interest. In recent years, for budgetary reasons, premature discharges may have become more common. The rise in the incidence of multiple admissions observed in recent years (13.9% in 1995 as compared with 12.1% in 1989) may well testify to this practice.

We conclude that the current medical system generally performs well in providing for financial accessibility. The concern is, rather, about ration, queues, and compromised quality of service.

Is Hong Kong's Medical Care System Burdensome?

Financial burden is different from *"financial accessibility"*. Whereas "feasible" means the absence of excessive hardship, "burden" refers to shouldering the economic cost, which need not imply hardship. Thus, a modest increase in burden that allows an improvement in quality may be desirable; but to achieve the same improvement with reduced financial accessibility is not desirable.

One simple measure of total burden is the total cost of the health care bill, regardless of how that burden is distributed between taxpayers, patients, and consumers of other government-provided services. It is the opportunity cost of the resources which are either expended directly on health care or indirectly as a result of diversion of resources from other uses into health care. A simple indicator of total burden is the percentage of the gross domestic product devoted to health care. Figures given in Table 1.5a and Table 1.5b show total health care spending and public spending on health care as a percentage of GDP.[6]

A more comprehensive measure of total burden should include the cost of avoidable inefficiency, including the time cost of patients and that of their family members in the waiting room. In general, time cost is reduced by the self-selection of patients. Patients with high values of time will generally not be attracted to the government clinics or the specialist clinics run by the Hospital Authority. However, even though the current system of health care is high in production efficiency, to the extent that consumers still lack autonomy over the quality of publicly provided health care services, there is inefficiency or *excess burden*. The following section turns to the question of financial burden.

Financial Burden

Conceptually, the total cost of the health care bill can be broken down in a number of different ways. The bill can be, for example, broken down by:

1. *Function*: direct patient care (primary, ambulatory care, acute and extended care), prevention, research and development, and medical education;
2. *Cost bearer*: private-borne cost, public-borne cost, costs borne by the present generation and costs borne by future generations; and
3. Cost *distinction*: between direct variable costs and overhead costs.

The decomposition of total cost by function is largely an allocative matter and relates to allocative efficiency. The breaking down of total cost by who bears the cost has to do with both relative and total burdens, while the distinction between variable costs and overhead costs has implications on pricing, if allocative efficiency is to be achieved.

According to the government's General Household Expenditure Survey done for 1994–95, the average percentage of (disposable) household income spent on medical services was only 1.23% for the 50% of households with monthly expenditures ranging from HK$4,000 to HK$15,999, and 1.62% for the 30% of households with monthly expenditures ranging from HK$16,000 to HK$29,999. Assuming a spending ratio of 1.5%, for a median income household in 1996 (HK$17,500 per month), health expenditures per year would amount to HK$3,150 if savings were zero. On the other hand, national income statistics suggest that per capita health consumption expenditures averaged HK$4,700 in 1995. While national income statistics and household expenditure survey statistics are based on different surveys and address different issues, a key explanation for the difference may be employer-paid health insurance or health benefits, which is considered health care expenditures in GDP statistics but is not covered in the General Household Survey.

Although these spending ratios suggest very low direct patient-borne burden, they may be misleading because things can be very much different for particular families when a major health problem strikes. In fact, it is over special circumstances that people are worried about. As discussed in the previous section, 34.8% of households sampled in the public survey in Hong Kong are worried or very much worried about unforeseen medical expenses, and as many as 54.8% of households indicated being "somewhat worried", "worried", or "very much worried".

How much more payment can families bear? Table 2.12 suggests that a large majority of households can spend up to 6% of their incomes on medical care without experiencing serious difficulties — far higher than the average spending ratios currently observed. Given that the entire HA budget for 1996–97 was HK$20.1 billion (HK$19,225 million allocation plus HK$141 million in other incomes plus HK$635 million from user charges), in per capita terms, the HA budget works out to about HK$3,190 per year, inclusive of patients' direct payment. For a typical household of three members, the average burden, if assigned to the household, would amount to HK$9,570 (HK$800 per month) or 4.6% of the median household income in 1996 (Table 2.14). Apparently, there is room for increasing burden without jeopardizing accessibility.

Making this observation is not the same as advocating the imposition of a health tax or a mandatory health insurance premium on Hong Kong's households. A discussion of reform options has to wait until Chapter 4, after a discussion of the theoretical issues in the next chapter. Here, merely the following should be noted:

1. In recent years taxpayers have been shouldering an ever larger burden of the total hospital care bill (including land and capital costs) both in absolute terms and relative to what is borne by patients.
2. Patients now bear about 3.17% of the total recurrent operating costs for Hong Kong's public hospitals and that the average direct burden on patients is by all measures very light, even though the burdens on particular patients may be much higher (Table 2.10).

3. Compared to public hospitals, private hospitals impose much higher charges (Table 2.15a); consequently, the burden on patients can be quite large. A vivid case study would demonstrate this point. Table 2.15b shows that for one patient, hospital charges, *excluding doctor's fees,* amounted to HK$17,918 for a five-day stay. Given the long queues of patients for most treatments and for some diagnostic procedures, some patients are forced into bearing the heavy burden of the cost of private hospital charges. It should be noted that the high charges notwithstanding, virtually all private hospitals are currently running deficits because of very high overhead costs.

Public Debate on Burden

A key question regarding burden is how burden is to be shared. Compared to direct charges on users of the health care system, tax financing is less visible because the taxes paid by a person are not directly related to the health services consumed. It is impossible to track down who shoulders, and how much he shoulders, the burden of, say, a million-dollar additional budget allocated to health care. Direct charges encourage economy and promote prevention. However, direct charges are also more regressive than taxes, partly because poorer people are more likely to have poorer health, and partly because, with taxes, particularly income taxes, it is possible to link payment with the ability to pay. With charges, to link payment with ability to pay is more difficult and administratively far more costly.

Given the lower visibility and higher progressivity of the burden of taxes, there is a tendency for community pressure groups to prefer taxes to direct charges. For example, the *Community Green Paper on Health Services* (1995), states, "The Government should

> ...Continue its policy of levying nominal charges for health services. Taxes, not charges, should be relied upon to finance health care costs.

...Increase expenditure on health care and upgrade the quality of health services.

...Set up an efficient mechanism for resource allocation and utilization in health care, announce to the public how such resources are being utilized, and delegate the responsibility of auditing to the Auditor-General's Office, so the Government may monitor closely how the Department of Health and the Hospital Authority functions.

...Gradually eliminate all itemized charges." (p. 41)

The opposite view is taken by the private hospitals who petitioned the government in the summer of 1996 to adopt a user-pays policy, with subsidization based on a means test. This was believed to be necessary in order for private hospitals to compete successfully with public hospitals. The community, however, must consider the risk of excessive burden that such a policy may imply. Based on the public survey results acquired, it is unlikely that there will be much support for such a policy.

Production Efficiency and Consumption Efficiency

Even though it is often thought that economists would recommend a user pays policy, tax financing of medical infrastructure is efficient and therefore consistent with least burden. In general, any item of medical infrastructure or equipment should be subject to benefit-cost analysis. When benefits are found to outweigh costs, it makes sense to rely on taxes to cover any shortfall of user fee revenue over costs, because efficient user fees should cover only marginal costs.

In principle, all health care costs can be broken down to two components: the overhead cost which does not vary with the number of patients serviced, and the variable cost which varies directly with the number of patients serviced. Users should pay for the full marginal cost of services because this is conducive to efficient utilization of the resources. If marginal costs happen to exceed average variable costs, pricing at marginal cost would lead to an operating surplus to contribute towards overhead costs. On the other hand, financing overhead cost generally with user fees may be excessively burdensome because charging fees above marginal cost would curtail consumption before marginal benefit falls to equate with marginal cost. This would be detrimental to consumption efficiency.

Consumption efficiency means that medical services and facilities are efficiently utilized to meet consumers' needs. In order to achieve this, prices should reflect marginal costs on the supply side, and consumer awareness of the true expected benefits of services on the demand side. The latter depends very much on the ability and the willingness of medical professionals to convey the expected benefits of services to patients and their families. In the context of asymmetric information and financial incentives of medical professionals to profit from services rendered, consumption efficiency cannot be guaranteed. Without denying that it could occur, it is entirely dependent on the professional ethics of doctors.

Production efficiency refers to the minimization of real resource input given the level of output, or to the maximization of output given the resource input. It says nothing about whether the factor inputs concerned are earning economic rent. If factor inputs are earning a large economic rent, the financial burden on those who pay for these inputs of course will be higher. But production may still be efficient. Production is efficient in so far as there are sufficient incentives for the real resources already committed to be put to the most productive use.

The inference that the current health care system is likely to be high in production efficiency is based on the budgetary arrangement of the Hospital Authority and the transparency of the budgetary processes. The Hospital Authority operates essentially on a principle of capitation. That is to say, the funding is based on a commitment to achieve certain service targets rather than being granted retroactively to tide over realized deficits. Even though the HA is funded by the government, it operates independently from the government and on a predetermined budget. Just as the HA is given its budget on the basis of a service agreement with the government, so the allocation of resources to hospitals for each year is based on the service agreement between the HA Head Office and hospitals. The budgetary and the annual planning processes are integrated to provide a mechanism to link resource inputs and budgets to service outputs, outcomes, and quality standards. For 1996–97, allocation to hospitals is based on three elements (see *Budget Allocation 1996/97*, Finance Committee, Hospital Authority):

1. *Baseline allocation*, which is largely based on the previous year's budget, taking into account the full year effect of the services introduced, adjustment for changes in service utilization, and net of the contributions for productivity gain. With this baseline allocation, each hospital promises to deliver services meeting targets in terms of volume, scope, and quality.

2. *Productivity gain initiatives*, which are assumed to release resources equal to 2.5% of the baseline budget. The released resources are redistributed for new and improved services.

3. *Specialty cost and patient-related groups* (PRGs), which applies to nine major acute hospitals and accounts for 30% of the 1996–97 baseline allocation. This allocation considers the special needs of hospitals providing special-ist services, while taking into account the expected caseload of patients falling into one of 13 PRGs, for each of which a data model has been developed describing the clinical management paths and the service profiles, and quantifying the key cost drivers.

Autonomy and Freedom of Choice

Autonomy is generally regarded as the hallmark of a profession and is an important basis for self-esteem. Health care professionals are also, by definition, more knowledgeable about the health care field than others. There is the presumption that they should know better than others what is best for patients. There is a firm belief within the profession that self-regulation and management by medical professionals is better than regulation by bureaucrats and management by nonmedical professionals. This is the main reason that a medical doctor was appointed to head the Hospital Authority and that a medical doctor occupies the important post of chairman of the Medical Council.

Table 2.16a and Table 2.16b show that generally more doctors regard professional autonomy in HA hospitals as "high" than those who regard such autonomy as "low", but there is a sizeable minority, well over 20%, who regard professional autonomy either as "low or very low". Moreover, autonomy is perceived to be much lower in HA hospitals than in non-HA hospitals in the minds of most doctors.

The effect of the budget constraint on professional autonomy is demonstrated in an incident cited in the *Ming Pao* (21 October 1996). According to this report, responding to a directive of the HA, Professor Jean Woo of the Department of Internal Medicine at the Chinese University of Hong Kong wrote an internal memorandum advising doctors in the Department of Internal Medicine in her hospital to prescribe low-cost medicines in order to avoid facing a cut in manpower. Specifically, she had reminded her colleagues to: use diuretics and betablockers for lowering blood pressure rather than calcium antagonists or ACE inhibitors; refer patients to the Outpatient Department as soon as they show signs of stabilizing conditions; prescribe medicines that are lowest in cost; avoid prescribing vitamins to patients month after month; and adhere to the prescription guide circulated recently.

Without disputing the need for some guidelines to remind doctors to prescribe drugs that are known to be more cost-effective, outright "delisting" of some drugs may cause unnecessary anxiety and patient resistance. According to Dr. Yip Wai Chun, then President of the Public Doctors Association, the policy of restricting the use of expensive drugs will have the largest impact on chronic patients, who will find it difficult to switch to a new drug when they have already been accustomed to another drug. He strongly defended doctors' autonomy in the prescribing of drugs. Moreover, controlling cost in contravention to doctors' autonomy and professional judgment may sometimes end up shifting costs rather than lowering costs. Premature discharging of patients and shifting patients to the Outpatient Department will lead to more frequent re-admissions, increasing the administrative burden in the Admissions Department and directly shifting costs to the Outpatient Department.

Conclusions

Hong Kong's publicly-funded health care system is generally of a quality that compares well with that of the private sector and is highly regarded by the public. The present system of health is also financially accessible. Indeed, financial accessibility is the predominant reason that a household would choose to use the HA system (Table 2.17). However, given the rapid ageing of the Hong Kong population, the constraint of the Basic Law on the tax system requiring Hong Kong to continue with a low tax rate regime, and the commitment of the Hong Kong government that public expenditures should not grow faster than the GDP, the publicly-funded health care system is facing increasing difficulty in keeping up with the same level of quality and accessibility, let alone improving quality.

The largest component in the Hospital Authority budget is personal emoluments (mainly salaries and wages), which account for 82% of recurrent spending. Doctors generally find the workload excessive, to the extent that quality of service may be jeopardized. Professional autonomy is generally lower in the HA hospitals than in private hospitals. However, doctors generally value greatly the opportunity to work in the HA establishment. The attrition rate in every category of workers, as Table 2.18 indicates, has fallen in recent years.

Compared to the publicly-funded health care sector, private health care services are much more expensive, but they are attractive because they offer savings in the time cost spent in queues; they offer faster treatment and diagnosis to avoid a loss in the opportunity of effective medical intervention; they offer greater autonomy; and they offer superior services for those who are willing to pay higher prices. However, the private hospital sector is grossly under-utilized. Notwithstanding much higher charges, most private hospitals, if not all, are running deficits.

Our survey in late 1996 indicated that respondents were willing to pay more taxes to get better health care services. Community pressure groups, however, are vocal in opposing greater reliance on fees paid by user. The survey shows that a significant minority of households are worried about excessive health care bills. The objection over itemized charges and user fees in general seems to be related to the uncertainty over the magnitude of the burden. In the next chapter, these and other issues will be examined in greater detail using tools of economic analysis.

Notes

1. In some jurisdictions, HMOs are required to take all enrollees and are given a direct lump-sum transfer from the government to enable them to meet costs that are commensurate with the demographic composition of the market population.

2. In terms of inpatient days, the share of private hospitals is much lower.

3. See the results of a public survey conducted by the author, which will be presented below.

4. For a philosophical discussion, see the section "Autonomy as Freedom" in Morreim (1995, Chapter 7).

5. Note that in the telephone interview the respondents are not prompted with respect to the reasons for preference.

6. These figures must be taken with caution. Noting the non-inclusion of the imputed rental values of buildings and facilities and the insufficient allowance for unpaid services offered by other government departments to the health sector, Hay (1992) estimated that "the actual levels (of public spending on health care) are conservatively double the Department of Health and Hospital Services Department budgets, and probably much larger than that."(p. 10)

CHAPTER 3

Economic Dimensions of Health Care and Principles in Health Policy

Introduction

This chapter explains the role of health in the economy and why it makes sense to devote more resources to health care when the economy develops and matures. It explains the nature of health policy, defines the players in the health equation, and explains the roles of each player. Finally, it analyzes the composition of health care cost and explains the role of benefit-cost analysis in the health care sector.

Why Health is of Value and Why Health Expenditures Should Rise

Health is valued by both households and employers. Health also fosters a sense of national pride. Households value health for its own sake and for the fact that it is an input in "household production" — the economist's jargon for household activities that contribute to utility. A state of excellent health also makes people feel good. Conversely, poor health makes people and their immediate family members feel bad.

Household production can be envisaged as the process of organizing and turning consumption goods and services purchased in the marketplace and other inputs into enjoyable, final objects of consumption such as a feeling of togetherness, the wonderful taste

43

of good food, relaxation, excitement and fun. One can envisage "healthy days" or "healthy time" as such an input. In the absence of healthy days or healthy time, it would be impossible to enjoy a picnic, a concert, a theatrical performance, a packaged tour, or a dinner party with friends and relatives. To take advantage of the good things offered by nature or modern science and technology, one has to be healthy.

Healthy days or healthy time is also an input in commercial production or social production. The lack of health lowers productivity and increases absenteeism.

The advent of modern science and technology has vastly increased the opportunities of consumption and production; so the value of health is also increasing by the day. Modern science and technology has raised the potential productivity of workers and has made available new goods and services that were formerly unthinkable. This has raised the opportunity cost of healthy days lost because of sickness. In general, if the opportunity cost of healthy days has gone up, more resources should be devoted to health, other things being equal.

Household Behaviour and the Social Demand for Health

One central assumption of economics is that human beings are rational. By this, economists mean that human beings and households behave in a consistent, predictable manner and can be assumed to maximize their perceived overall well-being, which is represented by an index called utility. Thus households maximize utility by adjusting their "decision variables" subject only to the constraints that may prevail at the time. Constraints include such things as the availability of goods and services in the marketplace, wages and prices, potential labour hours, information, and physical laws governing how the status of health changes with age, lifestyle, and health care inputs. One general theoretical setup is to assume that utility depends on (1) consumption variables which are produced through various household activities, (2) health status, and (3) time devoted to work. Households maximize utility by: allocating time between work that earns income and non-work activities; allocating time among various non-work activities which include socializing, entertainment, cultural activities, health care, sports and exercises, eating and so on; allocating income between savings and consumption; and allocating what is budgeted for consumption between health-related goods and services and other market goods and services, and also items within each of these categories of goods and services.

Policy Influence

Households engage in these maximizing activities in an environment that is largely external to them but one that is very much influenced by government policies. In four ways, health care of households is influenced by the government.

First, the household's after-tax income will depend on the tax rate, tax allowances, and transfer payments made by the government. Second, the prices of health care services are often either directly administered by the government or influenced substantially by the government. Third, the prices of products and services, the consumption of which have an impact on health, are also subject to influence by the government. Examples are alcoholic and tobacco products. Fourth, the availability of health care services, as well as the quality of such services, are subject to government discretion through its policy in providing various health care infrastructures as well as manpower. It must be noted that households do not have any control over these government policies in the short run, even though over time they may be able to influence the government to act one way or the other.

Households must take the physical laws which govern the changes of the health status as given. Thus, there are a number of things about health that households can do very little about. For example, households cannot prevent ageing from taking its toll on health, and they cannot drink excessively and be exempt from the consequences of excessive drinking. Households, however, can influence the health status by choosing their lifestyle. In particular, they can reduce consumption activities that are harmful to health, avoid excessive work or working in an environment that can damage health, avoid activities that are hazardous (such as car racing) or take precautions when they do engage in such activities. In the event that a health problem arises, households also have alternative courses of action. They can consult a doctor, take over-the-counter medications, take a rest, or simply ignore the problem. They must accept the consequences of their actions, whether they like it or not. In particular, they must recognize the fact that the better shape they keep themselves today, the better shape they will be in when they get up tomorrow.

One implication of this discussion is that while health is valued by households, and households do have a large degree of control over their health through their lifestyle and behaviour, they may not maximize health at all. To households, the benefit of better health in terms of direct contribution to utility, more healthy time, and thus greater potential for consumption, must be balanced against the sacrifice in terms of lost consumption opportunities and lost income. In particular, if the household "discounts" future utility greatly, then it is more likely that it may work or consume in a way that is detrimental to health. In general, households that are more unstable and those that live in a risky environment tend to have higher rates of discount. Members of such households attach less weight to promises of higher utility in the future because they may think that they may not live long enough to see the future. Thus, during times of war or in countries where there is a high risk of being killed, people tend to have a short time horizon. They will enjoy what they can today, without worrying about the consequences. Since bad health of high-risk households and individuals can increase the chances of the outbreak of epidemics, health care costs for the society in general can rise. So it is socially desirable to have more health (as a cushion) than the equilibrium amount of health that comes about as a result of households' maximizing behaviour. There is, clearly, a case for society to subsidize health care on grounds of efficiency.

Another implication of this discussion is that government policy has much influence on household behaviour, with consequences on both health and health care cost. A policy of imposing taxes on unhealthy consumption and providing subsidies on healthy activities will promote healthy lifestyles. A policy that shelters households from the cost of health care will encourage unhealthy lifestyles and will raise the cost of health care. While direct burden may be reduced by such policies, indirect yet real burden may explode, as has happened in a number of countries. A government that is successful in promoting political stability, in protecting citizens against crime, and in offering opportunities of growth and development will tend to extend the time horizon of households, leading to lower "discount rates", and will encourage households to choose a lifestyle healthier.

Efficient Production of Health

It is clear from the above that health is the joint outcome of private activity and public policy. In particular, public and private medical inputs are obviously substitutes. The more health care input is provided by the public sector, the less privately procured input will be needed. Within the public sector, medical inputs consist of inputs into health care infrastructure as well as recurrent inputs directly arising from health care of individuals. Within the private sector, households and health care providers interact, with consequences on health, and they interact in an environment that is determined by public policy. In particular, if the quality of publicly provided health care has improved, while charges remain the same or rise only slowly, then demand for private sector services will fall. In contrast, if the government requires everyone to subscribe to a health insurance plan that provides reimbursement for private sector services, the demand for private sector services will rise. Depending on the actual policy adopted, the budget constraint faced by the household will change, leading to a change in household behaviour and in the composition of health care services produced.

A key question is how to design a policy environment that will ensure that Hong Kong's health care services are produced efficiently. Putting it another way, the incentives of users and providers of medical services need to be structured in such a way that medical inputs are used efficiently in enhancing health. In this regard, the following ten peculiarities about health care must be noted.

Peculiar Aspects of Health Care

First, being consumers of health care services, households have very limited information on their own health status and the quality of health care provided by different physicians. Above all, households do not know what kind of health care services are most appropriate to their situations. Consumers of health care services generally depend on medical professionals to advise them about what treatment or diagnostic procedures are needed. Thus, here is a case of *information asymmetry*.

Second, even for professionals, obtaining updated, accurate information on patients may be quite costly. In a substantive sense, every patient is unique. Indeed, one could even argue that the situation of the same patient at any moment is unique. It is therefore necessary to deal with the problem of very high *information cost* in health care.

Third, medical expertise, drugs, and medical technology are all very expensive. With an ageing population, the cost of medical care is projected to continue to increase rapidly well into the future. This problem can be called *cost pressure–demographic pressure squeeze*.

Fourth, there are two kinds of medical care: chronic and episodic. Needs arising from chronic health problems are uninsurable in the private market because no insurer would offer a policy that is known to be money-losing. Indeed, someone with a known chronic health problem is not a *risk* to be insured against, but a *cost driver* to be dealt with.

Fifth, episodic health problems are insurable, but they are subject to the problem of moral hazard in the sense that insured people may take fewer preventive steps to avoid health problems (the so called consumer-side moral hazard), and that insured people are more likely to respond positively to medical doctors' advice for diagnostic procedures or treatment, which may be profit-motivated (producer-side moral hazard). It is now well known that third-party medical insurance with a fee-for-service policy tends to lead to explosive medical care expenditures. Insurers in the marketplace have generally responded to the problem with three measures to reduce insurers' liability: coinsurance requiring co-payment by patients for all marginal expenses, deductibles from total expenses, and reimbursement ceilings to cap claims. In addition, other market institutions have arisen to deal with the problem that doctors may not act in the best interest of patients and certainly not in the interest of insurers. In economics this is called the *principal–agent problem*. Doctors are the agents of households who are responsible for looking after their health. They are also the agents of insurance companies who have underwritten the health care costs of households, responsible for fulfilling the obligations of the insurance companies. Doctors, however, may not act in the interest of the principals.

Sixth, the *human capital investment problem* is an example of the principal–agent problem. In today's world, with rapidly changing technology and fast-accumulating knowledge, it is in the interest of consumers of health care services that medical professionals regularly update their knowledge. However, to the extent that consumers may not be able to tell if their doctors have the latest knowledge on treating their problems, doctors also may not have the incentive to acquire the skills. It is in the interest of doctors to acquire credentials that appear impressive and command a premium in the marketplace, but not in the interest of doctors to update or refresh their skills if patients cannot tell the difference. In a world of fee-for-service and imperfect information, time spent acquiring new skills or refreshing old skills may have a high opportunity cost in terms of income foregone but may not bring commensurate financial reward.

Seventh, medical insurance is subject to the *adverse selection problem*, which says that an insurance plan that offers a lot of protection tends to attract high risks, since it is too costly and unattractive for healthy individuals. It has been proved by economists that because of adverse selection, insurers are unlikely to profit from insurance plans that offer a lot of protection. This means that the average individuals who are risk averse are either unable to get the coverage they want or they have to pay an unattractively high premium for the protection.

Eighth, health care, whether of the preventive or the curative type, has *external effects* and *scale economies*. Thus, improved immunity against a disease achieved by injection of a vaccine among part of a population will benefit the rest of the population because other people's chances of contracting the disease will also come down. Moreover, the more people get immunized, the higher the cost-effectiveness of the immunization problem will be. Effectively curing a patient of tuberculosis will also reduce the chances of the disease spreading to other people.

Ninth, while there are random factors that affect health, many of these "random" factors are actually traceable to the *behaviour of individuals*. Thus, more drunk drivers on the road would increase the unfavourable ("random") chance for traffic accidents which adversely affect the general health of the population. The outbreak of an epidemic may be traceable to some individual's failure to observe common sense hygiene.

Finally, some health care expenditures are known to relate to the phenomenon of *defensive medicine*. One cause of the health cost explosion in the United States has been traced to physicians administering normally unnecessary diagnostic tests and medications to ward off malpractice suits. Clearly, defensive medicine has no place in a world of efficient production of health care services. According to two Stanford University economists, Daniel Kessler and Mark McClelland (*Business Week* 13 May 1996), "defensive medicine has been a widespread and costly practice, one that could be reduced through liability reforms." These economists analysed hospital expenditures for all elderly Medicare patients hospitalized in 1984, 1987, and 1990 with recently diagnosed heart attacks and other serious heart ailments. Controlling various factors in the

Table 3.1

Decline in Job-related Health Insurance Coverage in the U.S., 1979 and 1992

Educational Background	1979 (%)	1992 (%)
High school dropouts	88	54
High school graduates	89	68
Some college	86	72
College graduates	86	75
All workers	87	70

Source: *Business Week,* 21 August 1995.

analysis, they discovered that reforms that resulted in limiting liability awards had reduced growth rates of hospital outlays noticeably — lowering them by as much as 5% to 9% compared to states with no reforms. This was achieved without noticeable effect on the health of patients. The authors estimated that nationwide comprehensive limits on malpractice awards could reduce annual health care outlays by up to $50 billion.

The Distributional Aspects of Health Policy

"[I]t is hard to have reform without also having substantial redistribution." So wrote Joseph Newhouse in the opening article for Symposium on Health Care Reform in The *Journal of Perspectives* (1994). While intended to apply to the American case, what Newhouse wrote applies with equal force to the case of Hong Kong.

The fact that health policy has a significant impact on distribution is apparent from the sheer size of health care expenditures relative to the gross domestic product. Significantly, while an ill-conceived health policy can have perverse distributional effects, an enlightened health policy will have desirable redistributional consequences compared to the status quo. Jane Sneden of the Federal Reserve Bank of Boston, in an article cited in *Business Week* (21 August 1995), wrote: "In no other high income country has the growing cost of health care contributed to rising earnings inequality as it has in the U.S." Because of health insurance cost inflation, over the years, more and more of the less educated Americans were denied health insurance (Table 3.1). This had contributed to a real decline in the take-home pay of the less educated. A health policy that extends health insurance to those in marginal employment and to the unemployed will generally redistribute in favour of the poor.

The redistributive consequences of health policy are not only limited to vertical effects, but they may also cut across different industries and occupations in a way that may not be vertically systematic. In particular, health policy redistributes among: different interest groups such as health care service providers, insurers, lawyers, and consumers; different demographic groups, particularly the elderly, who are more likely to be chronically ill; different categories of taxpayers who may be subject to different tax increases or decreases on account of a change in health policy; and different categories of consumers of government services which could be cut to different extents in order to make way for health care spending.

Although the redistributive effects of health policy are real, redistributive effects should not be confused with the award of benefits under an insurance system. An insurance system that pools premiums together and awards benefits to policy subscribers is not redistributive in the traditional sense of the word. An insurance system is redistributive if and only if the premiums of some classes of subscribers are subsidized up front by other subscribers.

The potential redistributive effects of health policy may well have potent effects on resource allocation. For example, in a regime of mandatory health insurance with employers being held responsible for the premiums, a payroll tax to pay for the premiums with a cap on total contributions will favour high-wage firms relative to low-wage firms, compared to a regime that caps contributions attributed to individuals (Cutler, 1994, pp. 25–26). These discriminatory effects between high-wage and low-wage firms will have implications on the relative profitability of different sectors and hence on investment.

The Validity and Necessity of Benefit-Cost Analysis in Health Care Analysis

It must be stressed that, in the final analysis, optimal policy design can only be based on benefit-cost analysis of alternative policy options, and optimal health care outlay can only be based on benefit-cost analysis of alternative outlays. It is often held that health and life are not market commodities and should not carry price tags. Many people believe that "life is priceless" with the implication that any amount of money should be spent as long as lives are saved. It is important to see the flaw in such arguments. Benefit and cost calculations will be necessary as long as resources are scarce and intelligent choices need to be made about the use of resources. As long as choices have to be made, the ranking of alternatives is unavoidable. Benefit and cost calculations merely represent a way of indexing alternatives in a consistent fashion so that alternatives can be ranked and choices made.

Without downplaying the respect for life, putting "price tags" on lives saved or risked is necessary because otherwise policy decisions will be made arbitrarily. There is no basis to judge the relative superiority of alternative policy options. It is important to note that "saving lives" in fact means, at the most, extending lives. Lives can never be saved forever because death is inevitable. Extending a life for a longer time is presumably worth more than extending a life for a shorter time, other things being equal. In real life, however, "other things" are typically not equal. Diverting resources to save one life will either lead indirectly to other people having shorter lives, or to other people having lower-quality lives. The benefit of saving or extending one life must therefore be compared with the cost before determining if the extension is worthwhile.

Economists value lives by adding up the values of surviving years. The values of surviving years comprise expected productivity and the value of household activities made possible by survival. In principle, one could add the moral values that an individual and other members of the society place on one person's survival. Even though these values are difficult to impute, they must not be assumed infinite; otherwise, rational decision making would be impossible.

In recent years the concept of quality-adjusted life years (QALYs) has come into vogue. The concept is a logical derivative from the intuition that a year of survival with a high quality of life must be worth more than a year of survival with a lower quality of life. Intelligent comparison will require translating different quality life-years into equivalent (quality-adjusted) life-years. Thus one "quality X" life-year may be worth k times more than one "quality Y" life-year, where "k" is a translation factor (or a relative worthiness factor) to be estimated. A unified way of converting dissimilar objects into comparable units is to use shadow prices to value or determine the cost of those objects. Shadow prices are so called because they cannot be observed in the market place and must be imputed.

To illustrate the concept in a more practical context, consider the medical procedures that extend patients' lives while inflicting discomfort or, alternatively, medical procedures that shorten patients' lives while reducing discomfort. The concept of QALY is to allow us to evaluate and compare the desirability of such procedures and practices. One approach is to use the following model in evaluating the output of a medical procedure.

In the case where life is extended, the value of the procedure can be calculated by a formula [1] and compared to the value for the alternative case where life is shortened.[2]

In the above the comparison of the two values presumes that there exists a ready "shadow price" for life-years of a given quality. Clearly this is a simplification used only to illustrate the trade-off between length of life and quality of life. In practice it will be necessary to consider the many dimensions of quality of life such as mobility, ability to communicate, sense of touch, taste, sight, hearing, and self-care ability, and price the separate dimensions separately. Pain and discomfort should be priced negatively. There is moreover a personal valuation of one's own life that may be independent of the above (e.g. the moral value). For example, consider an individual who have a strong will to live notwithstanding pain and loss of most faculties. The value of a life of any normal person in principle can be calculated.[3] We can likewise calculate the respective values of a disease-handicapped life-year and that of a rehabilitated life-year.[4]

In this manner of valuation of QALYs, the relative merits of various medical procedures, and by extension, that of various health policies can be conducted (at least numerically if not objectively). Such are the quantitative contributions of health economics to policy evaluation. Beyond quantitative considerations, moreover, health policies must observe certain economically and ethically sound principles in order that net benefits are maximized and distributed fairly among population groups. In the next section, five such "Principles" in health policy are described.

Principles in Health Policy

These five principles should be observed in devising health policies that seek an optimal balance of competing demands. In Chapter 2, an example of competing demand can be found in "three-way trade-offs" among quality, accessibility, and burden.

Principle One: Optimal Allocation of Resources into Health Care

Quality of health care and financial accessibility to health care should be increased as long as the benefits as perceived by the community are larger than the cost of the resources involved in terms of the sacrifice of other socially desirable goods and services.

The total amount of resources allocated to health care in many countries is a result of both public and private decision making. Within the public sector it is determined through a budgetary process which may be highly political, involving a change in taxes collected or a revision in the order of priority vis-a-vis other government-provided services. Within the private sector it is determined in the marketplace through the interaction of producers and consumers of health care services.

Some countries have chosen to cap the total amount of public funds provided for health care. Within the total budget defined by the cap and made available for health care, medical professionals seek to maximize the total output or value of health care services. To some extent, such caps give the government some protection from ongoing political pressure to increase public spending on health care.

Governments generally have a large impact on how much is allocated privately on health care. The regulatory environment, in particular laws relating to advertising and insurance, will influence how much is spent on health care within the private sector.

Given the total resources allocated to health care, three questions immediately follow. The first question pertains to the sharing of the burden among members of society. Society will seek the optimal sharing of burden, the meaning of which will be explored shortly. Another question pertains to the optimal allocation of health care resources for different aspects of health care. Of particular interest is the allocation between preventive medicine and treatment. The third question, referred to earlier, is whether to provide basic care to more people (more accessibility to basic care), or more *quality* care to some people selected on the basis of a particular criteria (for example, first come, first served).

Principle Two: Optimal Balance between Prevention and Treatment

Resources should be allocated to preventive medicine as long as the benefit is greater than that arising from devoting the same resources to treatment.

Principle Three: Optimal Balance between Financial Accessibility and Quality

Resources should be allocated to improve financial accessibility as long as the social benefit is greater than that arising from devoting the same resources to enhancing quality.

One way of looking at the question of how to divide the burden of financing health care is to consider that three groups jointly finance the provision of health care, namely, health care service users, taxpayers, and users of non-health care government services. Users can pay directly when they use the health care services, or they can pay for the use of such services by subscribing to a health insurance scheme. Taxpayers contribute to the financing of health care when general tax revenue is used to finance publicly provided health care services. Finally, health care services may be financed by cutting back other public services.

The principle of least burden says that the burden of providing for health care services should be allocated among taxpayers (who pay taxes), non-taxpayers (who may suffer a decline in the quality of some public services), and health care service users (who may have to pay fees, insurance premiums, or suffer a decline in the quality of medical services) in such a way that the cost to society is minimized. This means that if the social cost of assigning $1 of burden to patients is lower than the social cost of assigning $1 of burden to taxpayers, the cost should be assigned to patients. It also means that if the social cost of assigning $1 of burden to patient A is higher than that of assigning it to patient B, the burden should be assigned to B rather than to A. Finally, it further requires that if the social cost of cutting $1 of health care spending is lower than the social cost of cutting $1 of education spending, health care spending should be cut. Conversely, if the social cost of cutting $1 of health care spending is higher than that of cutting $1 of education spending, that one dollar should be allocated to health care services rather than education services.

In recent years there has been much discussion about the user-pays principle. It is widely believed, and economists are reputed to uphold, that making users pay for what they consume is both equitable and efficient. Actually such a belief is misplaced. The user-pays principle is valid only *at the margin*. That is to say, if users consume more of a service, they should pay for the cost of the services thus used up. If they are not willing to pay for the service, then presumably the cost is higher than the value of the service. The resources involved should be saved for alternative uses. Since most public services involve many fixed costs, there is a difference between users paying for margin costs and users paying for total costs. In general, marginal costs are much lower than average costs. If users had to pay for the *average* cost of everything, they would reduce their demand drastically — they would refrain from using a service even if the marginal benefit is higher than the marginal cost. Many facilities would be underutilized. The society would end up not having the benefit of those facilities and services at all.

Suppose university students had to pay for the full average cost of university education, patients had to pay for that of hospital services, passengers had to pay for that of the mass transit system, and motorists had to pay for that of roads and highways. All of these services would end up under-utilized because of the much higher fees, leading to gross inefficiency and waste.

In general, then, in the interest of efficiency, subject to the government's being able to finance the overhead costs, users of various public services should only pay for the marginal cost. One complication and caveat is that taxes generally have to be raised in order to meet the high fixed-costs requirements; yet, taxes are costly to raise too, involving collection costs, compliance costs, and above all, distortion costs — the costs of distorting the behaviour of consumers, wage earners and investors. So economists do talk about "optimal deviations from marginal cost pricing" (Baumol and Bradford, 1970). In any case, there is a clear case for sharing costs between users and taxpayers.

Principle Four: The Least Burden Principle

Least burden is achieved when the marginal cost of a health dollar raised from taxes, the marginal cost of a dollar paid in health care fees, and the marginal cost of a dollar transferred from alternative uses into health care in terms of the value foregone, are equalized.

To the extent that distributive concerns and accessibility do matter in health policies, optimal sharing of burden should also involve considerations of equity and ability to pay. For the poor, paying for the marginal cost of health care services may still be too much — unless there is a transfer that raises their ability to pay. Otherwise, in order that they have access to health care services, there is a case for allowing them to pay less than the marginal cost — in any case, to pay less than higher-income households.

Principle Five: Discount for the Poor Principle

Unless there are transfers to the poor, one could make a case for subsidizing marginal health care costs expended on the poor.

Conclusions

Health is the outcome of the interaction of various parties including households, health care givers, the government, and insurance companies. Health policy determines the way these parties relate to one another, their budget constraints, and their incentives. The challenge of health care policy design is to work out the benefit and cost implications of alternative policy options, in all the relevant dimensions, so as to choose the best that meet society's needs.

Notes

1. The value of a medical procedure in the case that life is extended *equals* to the change in value of each year of life as a result of the procedure *plus* the value of additional life-years after the procedure. Literally, the formula is:

   Sum over i (shadow price of a life-year at quality-after-procedure *minus* shadow price of life-year at quality-before-procedure) for year i, for all years of expected remaining life without the procedure
   plus
   Sum over j (shadow price of a life-year at quality-after-procedure) for year j up to expected end of life with the procedure.

2. As in [1] for the case where life is shortened, the value of the medical procedure *equals* to the change in value of each year of life as a result of

the procedure up to expected end of life with the procedure *minus* the value of life wiped out by the procedure. Literally:

Sum over i (shadow price of a life-year at quality-after-procedure *minus* shadow price of life-year at quality-before-procedure) for year i up to expected end of life with the procedure

minus

Sum over j (shadow price of a life-year at quality-before-procedure) for year j up to expected end of life without the procedure.

3. Value of a normal life is calculated by the formula which is, literally:

Sum over i (normal quantity measure of life faculty i *times* unit shadow price of life faculty i),

minus Cost of Pain,

plus Personal Moral Value of Life.

4. Value of a disease-handicapped life-year (affliction A) or that of a rehabilitated life-year (condition B) can be respectively calculated by the literal formula:

Sum over i (quantity measure of life faculty i under affliction A, or rehabilitated condition B *times* unit shadow price of life faculty i),

minus Cost of Pain in Condition A or Condition B,

plus Personal Moral Value of Life.

CHAPTER 4

The Available Policy Options

Introduction

As shown in the Chapter 3, a good health care system should be able to solve several problems in order to arrive at a solution that would balance the competing needs from the producers and suppliers. This chapter classifies these problems into five areas for which policy options are presented. The first is the *moral hazard* problem of the consumers of health care. The solution lies in preserving incentives for prevention of illnesses or injury. The second problem is also related to moral hazard but on the suppliers' side. The solution lies in preserving incentives for health care providers to deliver services in the interest of consumers while minimizing costs *(the principal agent problem)* even though information cost makes it difficult to monitor if they indeed do so. Besides, we need to compensate health care providers sufficiently for human capital investment, so that the necessary number of skilled personnel will be available to man the system *(human capital investment problem)*. The third problem, *risk management*, should be dealt with by providing affordable insurance against risks of catastrophic expenses arising from normal care in the event of serious illness or injury. The fourth is a *freedom of choice* problem which calls for allowing freedom of choice to opt for state-of-the-art care by paying more, either through direct payment or through extra insurance premiums. The fifth problem is concerned with *equity* issues. On the one hand, the health care system should offer a financing system that includes fees, insurance premiums, taxes, and possible cutbacks of other existing public services *(least burden)* and allows the optimal allocation between health care and non-health care needs. On the other hand, the system should allow equitable sharing of cost *(equitable sharing of burden)*. Policy options and the concrete arrangements for dealing with these problems will be discussed in turn.

The Moral Hazard Problem (Consumer Side)

General Discussion

Moral hazard (consumer side) is the phenomenon of insured persons taking fewer precautions or preventive actions to ward off potential risks, and of insured persons abusing health care services because they are sheltered from the full cost of the covered services.

Moral hazard in the form of reduced preventive effort is an aspect of rational behaviour, because while precautionary or preventive actions involve the same marginal costs independently of whether one is insured, insurance has reduced the expected benefit of those precautionary or preventive actions. To alleviate the problem, it is necessary to increase the expected marginal benefit of precautionary or preventive actions.

Policy Options

To deal with the problem of moral hazard of consumers, private insurers would reimburse only a percentage of the medical costs for each consultation ("coinsurance"). Alternatively, policies may require that patients pay costs up to a stated amount (a "deductible"). Such arrangements will reinstate some of the incentives for preventive actions which otherwise may be reduced as a result of the insurance policy.

From the public policy point of view, making households responsible for part or all of health care costs is necessary in order to deal with the moral hazard problem. There are two approaches to doing this. The first approach is to adopt the user pays principle with at least partial cost recovery for services rendered, so as to increase the out-of-pocket cost of falling sick. The second is to cap the quality of publicly funded services available, so as to increase the cost of falling sick in terms of discomfort.

Both approaches are effective. In the extreme, by definition, under unlimited full-cost recovery, there is no consumer-side moral hazard. Similarly, if the quality of services available through subsidized health care agents is capped at zero, consumers will have to be responsible for the full cost of health care to be provided in the private sector. Both approaches, however, carry potentially very high costs.

The first approach increases the financial risks of households and potentially jeopardizes the accessibility to health care services. The second approach penalizes households which, through no fault of their own, require medical services of a certain quality that is now made unavailable in order to head off moral hazard. In practice, however, judicious utilization of both approaches are necessary in an efficient health care system. That is, households must pay, and quality must be limited. Two key questions are then in order: How much households should pay, and how quality is to be limited.

In Singapore as well as in Hong Kong, the quality of subsidized health care is capped. Both systems promise to provide medical attention in the subsidized wards that is not unequal to that offered in the far more expensive private wards. However, these wards provide much less privacy, and patients accommodated therein are much more likely to be disturbed. Subsidized wards are also generally less spacious and provide fewer amenities (Class C ward in Singapore and public wards in Hong Kong) compared to private wards, which are not subsidized.

In Hong Kong, with the cost difference between subsidized wards and private wards rising, with the commitment to make health care equally accessible to patients of all wards, and with the quality of public wards rising, private wards have become less and less attractive. With the exception of the very rich, senior civil servants, and those who have insurance coverage, the greater majority of patients now opt for the heavily subsidized public wards. This has led to cost pressure as well as a failure of the system to ward off consumer-side moral hazard. Households have become less interested in adopting a healthy lifestyle.

To reinstate the incentives for households to adopt a healthier lifestyle, patients may have to pay higher charges for services rendered. Alternatively, the quality of subsidized health care could be reduced. The latter approach, however, seems undesirable and politically infeasible if it implies unequal access to medical attention.

In order not to jeopardize the principle of financial accessibility, there is a case for either capping the financial responsibility of households, or availing the households of a source of financing that can be spent on health care. Singapore has adopted the latter approach. The Medisave plan is a compulsory savings scheme capturing 6% to 8% of an individual's monthly income (depending on age) into a personal account from which medical bills can be paid. There are three disadvantages to this approach. One disadvantage is that large medical expenses may have to be incurred before the funds build up sufficiently. There is pressure for the government to assist when this happens, and provisions may have to be made for the government to take up this responsibility. Another disadvantage is that, as a compulsory scheme, it is insensitive to individual circumstances and preferences. It is paternalistic and may be resented by individuals who believe in freedom of choice. Finally, a Medisave plan may actually be ineffective as a way to promote preventive behaviour. To the extent that individuals have been forced to stock up large savings which can only be spent on medical expenses, there will be less incentive to adopt a healthy lifestyle. With less money available to be spent on non-health expenses, health actually may become less valuable.

This general discussion suggests that to contain moral hazard on the consumer-side, making households responsible for their own medical expenses up to some limit per year may be a sensible way to induce a healthy lifestyle; this way, financial accessibility to health care would not be compromised.

The Moral Hazard Problem (Producer Side)

General Discussion

The moral hazard problem on the producers' side is tricky because of the very high information cost in ascertaining actual behaviour of the health care providers and the various kinds of agents, for example, insurance agents or general practitioners who refer cases to specialists. Practice in the medical professions requires specialized knowledge and training. It is very difficult for someone without sufficient background to judge whether a medical doctor has made a reasonable judgement in a particular case or has made an error that should not have been made. There are two aspects of this moral hazard problem: the principal–agent problem and the human capital investment problem.

To deal with the principal–agent problem, there are two alternative approaches. The first is to design a contract between the principal and the agent that aligns the interest of the principal and that of the agent, so that the agent's self-interest corresponds with the principal's interest. The other is to hand out penalties or rewards according to the performance or behaviour of the agents as assessed through a monitoring mechanism. Because of the high cost of monitoring, typical policy responses are variants of the first approach. The general idea is to remove the opportunity for health caregivers to profit from activities that are against the interest of the principals — the patient or the insurer.

Policy Options

In the case of caregivers serving as insurers' agents, an example of the first approach is a system of prospective payment that links pre-specified lump sum payments to different diagnostic groupings (Diagnostic Related Groups or DRGs[1]). The insurer no longer pays the health care provider sums on demand on the basis of services performed. The health care provider, typically a hospital, will have the incentive to avoid unnecessary costs because it will collect surplus over the caring costs. This arrangement deals effectively with the principal–agent problem between the insurer and the health care provider so that the health care provider will have an incentive to minimize costs.

Still, in the absence of other provisions to protect the interest of the patient, DRGs are unsatisfactory in that they fail to deal with the principal–agent problem between the patient and the health care provider. A hospital will have the incentive to minimize care, possibly to the detriment of the interest of the patient.

A Health Maintenance Organization (HMO) is more satisfactory in this regard. It provides a prepayment system that combines the health insurance function with health care delivery. It takes care of people enrolled in the HMO programme. Because its profit is based on the revenue derived from attracting enrollees (who must pay the contract price to enrol) minus the cost of the medical attention given these enrollees, HMOs have both the incentive to achieve quality (so that they can draw enrollees) and the incentive to minimize costs (so that they can maximize the surplus).

HMOs, however, do have some serious drawbacks. For one thing, HMOs would not voluntarily and knowingly take on an enrollee if he or she has a chronic health problem that is costly to deal with. As HMOs would prefer that such people do not enrol, they do not need to provide quality services to attract them. Instead, they have every incentive to reduce the level of care since reducing the level of care will save costs and will discourage the undesirable enrolment. Another problem is that while HMOs want to give the impression that they provide good services to enrollees, the actual quality of services may nevertheless be questionable. In a recent issue of *USA Today* (18 December 1996), it was reported that U.S. HMOs were trying hard to reassure consumers that their plans were fair and transparent. To ward off regulations and rules by the federal government in protection of consumers' interest, the American Association of Health Plans (AAHP), which covers 87% of the 160 million Americans enrolled in managed care plans, wants its members to give more and better information about how their doctors are paid, why care is sometimes denied, and what specific prescriptions are covered; it has urged members to provide enrollees a choice of doctors.

One way to strengthen the incentive of HMOs to care for their enrollees is to require HMOs to underwrite a life insurance policy for each of their enrollees. It does not matter if this underwriting is subcontracted to other insurers in the market because market insurers will charge higher premiums if the HMO has a poor record of caring for its members and therefore more deaths among them. If the HMOs underwrite the lives of enrollees on their own, then a low quality of care leading to a higher incidence of death will hurt profits.

Following the same logic, if patients admitted into HA hospitals assessed not to be suffering from a critical condition have the option to buy a standard term life insurance policy from the hospital while being under its care, the incentive to provide better care will be enhanced.

As explained in Chapter 2, the publicly provided health care system in Hong Kong is like a giant HMO that covers all Hong Kong belongers. Because enrolment is by default, the problem of not covering chronic patients does not arise. As both insurer and caregiver at the same time, the Hospital Authority (HA) has incentive to provide effective, low cost services. Medical professionals employed by the HA are paid salaries and do not have an incentive to oversupply services. This is quite different in the case of fee-for-service arrangements, under which doctors need to have a high standard of professional ethics to avoid profiting from unnecessary services. Such a high standard of professional ethics is of course highly desirable but cannot be taken for granted. Indeed, anecdotal evidence suggests that some doctors affiliated with private hospitals do provide unnecessary services to enhance income.[2]

While compensation by salary rather than by fee-for-service will avoid some of the supply-side moral hazard effect, the level of compensation itself may affect efficiency and is certainly an important matter of public policy. In this regard, modern economics has some insight to offer. The theory of efficiency wages says that a low level of wages may depress morale. Increasing wages from such a level will induce effort and elicit better performance. As nominal wages increase, the cost per efficiency unit of work will decline up to a point, beyond which the cost will increase. Beyond the efficient wage any performance enhancement will lag behind the wage increase so that the wage increase will not be worthwhile to the employer.

The medical profession being a life career, the theory of efficiency wage must be adjusted. In order to enhance the junior medical doctor's desire to invest in career development and to reduce monitoring cost, a backloaded or deferred compensation profile may be adopted. That is to say, the salary may start from a low point — well below the actual value of the doctor's services — and end at a high point that is well above the value of the doctor's services. The potential salary increases give stronger incentive for the doctor to avoid being caught negligent (thus reducing monitoring cost) and to train to acquire better skills (so that he will qualify for promotion or move to a higher salary point).

While a fee-for-service type of compensation package to doctors may bias incentives towards oversupply of services, a fee-for-service setup may improve efficiency if the fees are set only to recoup direct costs. To the extent that such a level of a fee will not enhance the economic well-being of service providers, supply-side moral hazard may be contained. As patients are charged directly for costs expended, demand-side moral hazard may also be contained since households may want to reduce their need for health care services by adopting a healthier lifestyle.

The concept of HMOs as a team of health care professionals given the responsibility to look after the health of their enrollees and championing their health care interest is an extremely attractive one. Given the professional knowledge of their medical teams, HMOs are in a good position to serve as advocates for their enrollees if the enrollees require services provided by other medical service suppliers. A similar idea was promoted by a British health economist Alan Maynard, who championed the case of the family doctor serving as the patient's advocate to buy needed hospitalization services if required. By the same token, it is possible to envisage an HA doctor serving as the advocate of a patient under his care even though the patient may be referred to caregivers outside the HA system. Given the excessive utilization rates of public hospitals and the excess capacity of private hospitals, it is socially desirable if HA doctors who have more patients than they are capable of caring for can refer them to the private sector. They can help monitor the delivery of services by private doctors for their patients. This will reduce moral hazard and save costs.

The Human Capital Investment Problem

The human capital investment problem is another aspect of the principal agent problem on the supply side. In the face of imperfect information, doctors operating in a fee-for-service environment have little incentive to upgrade their skills unless those skills are easily recognizable by their patients and are rewarded. On the other hand, if doctors are salaried and their performance is assessed by their peers for promotion or career development purposes, the incentive to receive training will be higher. In any case, most likely they will be paid while attending training. In contrast, in a fee-for-service environment, the training can involve very high opportunity cost, and it may not bring financial rewards.

Over the long run, whether there is a steady and adequate supply of medical professionals depends on whether the return to human capital investment is sufficiently attractive. In general, there is a need to control the number and the quality of medical professionals to be supplied over some time horizon; and there is a need to continually upgrading the knowledge and skills of the existing stock of health professionals. As stressed earlier, consumers are not in the position to judge the professional ability of doctors, nurses, technicians, and pharmacists because of lack of knowledge and because of heavy information cost. Given the heavy cost incurred in the training of these professionals, it is important that only those with the right preparation and the right motivation enter the profession. It is necessary to maintain high standards throughout the training and provide graduates with a sufficient and relatively low-risk rate of return to human capital investment in order to draw potential devoted professionals into this challenging career.

Risk Management

General Discussion

It is reasonable to assume that all human beings are averse to large risks. That is to say, if there is a risk for a major disaster, human beings would be prepared to pay a premium to insure against that risk even if the cost of insurance is actuarially biased against him.

There are primarily two approaches to risk management. The first is the "saving for a rainy day" approach. Each individual would save a portion of his income each period and thus would accumulate a fund from which resources could be drawn in case of exigencies. The second is the "risk-pooling" approach. Different individuals would contribute an amount which will be pooled together. In the event a disaster strikes, resources can be drawn from the common pool to meet the needs of individuals facing exigencies.

There are both merits and demerits in each approach. The merit of the saving-for-a-rainy-day approach is that moral hazard is less of a problem. With each individual accountable entirely to oneself, people are less likely to relax their efforts to prevent the occurrence of exigencies. However, if the savings are forced, and the forced savings are earmarked only for health care, the problem could still surface. Another problem is that the accumulated savings of the individual simply may not be enough, and that with each person left to deal with his own problems alone, a larger savings on average will be required in order to provide a margin of comfort. There is also an absence of a feeling of mutual support, which may be valued for its own sake.

The merit of the risk-pooling approach is that there is a feeling of mutual support whenever disaster strikes anyone and that the insurance premium is likely to be smaller than the savings required under the saving for a rainy day approach. However, there is a larger risk of moral hazard. Insured individuals are likely to make less effort to prevent the occurrence of the insured event because such efforts yield less expected gain once the event has been insured.

Policy Options

The National Health Plan of Singapore, as unveiled in February 1983, introduced a "Medisave" scheme which is modelled under the saving-for-the-rainy-day approach (Kwa 1996). Under this scheme, a Medisave account is set up in the Central Provident Fund for medical expenses both for the account holder and for his or her family. However, the plan also incorporates some elements of risk pooling. Class C beds in government hospitals, in particular, are subject to large government subsidies. Government-subsidized beds, like explicit medical insurance schemes, represent risk pooling to the extent that beneficiaries draw from a common pool of funds into which people contribute as taxpayers. People are "insured" to the extent that they pay less than full costs when they need hospitalization.

Whichever approach towards risk management for health care service consumers is adopted, it is important to note that the bottom line is that consumers do not want to be caught in a situation where they have to face, unexpectedly, a bill that preempts the normal consumption of other goods and services and thus causes them great hardship. Ultimately, a health care scheme must be judged against the criterion of being able to protect consumers against unexpected, large outlays that will cause great hardship.

From this basic requirement, it is possible to envisage a variant of the risk-pooling or insurance approach. A cap can be placed on the total health care expenses of a household in any given year. This is related to catastrophe insurance. Singapore, in 1990, introduced a "Medishield" scheme to supplement the Medisave scheme. It is designed to help members meet heavy medical expenses arising from major or prolonged illnesses. It works like a typical insurance scheme, requiring the payment of an insurance premium, and qualifying the benefits with copayments and deductibles. The Medishield plan, unlike Medisave, is not compulsory, but 87% of Medisave members subscribed to it. The majority of those who opted out of Medishield already enjoy generous medical benefits from their employers or are covered by other plans. In addition to the 1.5 million Medisave members who subscribed to Medishield, some 240,000 dependents also joined. The Singapore experience shows that the demand for protection against large, unforeseen health expenditures is universal. A medical care scheme that does not provide for this type of insurance is unsatisfactory.

Apart from the need to manage risks for consumers of health care services, insurers and health care service providers also have to manage their own risks. For insurers, it has been noted that offering a plan that offers more coverage tends to attract higher risks — a phenomenon known as "adverse selection". Insurers either have to offer plans that protect less or have to charge premiums that would disadvantage those who belong to the normal-risk class. Since very costly policies will mainly attract high-risk subscribers and not enough low-risk subscribers, the typical market response of the insurance companies to the problem of adverse selection is the setting up of claim-caps — by limiting the claims that can be made. Table 4.1 shows the premiums chargeable for different clients for a Blue Cross medical insurance plan which carries a maximum benefit of US$250,000. Another approach is group insurance. Group insurance is the insurers' approach in screening out high-risk subscribers or at least in enlisting low-risk subscribers along with high-risk ones. Mandatory insurance is a special case of group insurance designed to deal with the same problem.

Not only do consumers and insurers face risks. Health care service providers also have to deal with risks. Their main risk lies in being sued and convicted for malpractice. The high cost of health care in the United States is at least partly due to the high cost of malpractice insurance. As discussed earlier, this situation has improved noticeably over the last few years, even though in the past the average medically related court award had gone up significantly and caused a run-up in costs. Average medical malpractice awards

Table 4.1
Premiums of Blue Cross Medical Insurance
(US$)

Age Group	Male	Female
0–17	823	823
18–25	1,124	1,462
31–45	1,371	1,783
46–50	1,508	1,961
51–55	1,645	2,139
56–60	1,824	2,261
61–65	2,098	2,601

Source: *Ming Pao*, 5 December 1996.
Note: Benefits amount to US$ 550 per day up to a yearly maximum of US$ 250,000 in compensation for hospitalisation, surgery, and incidental fees.

had increased from US$229,000 in 1975 to US$888,000 in 1983 and then to over US$1,000,000 in 1985 (Stoline and Weiner 1993, p. 205). The risks have suddenly become so high that several major companies which had been offering malpractice insurance quitted this market; and that those remaining have raised premiums dramatically. Some states have begun to limit the amount of the awards. As was pointed out in Chapter 3, the latest development is that American health cost inflation has abated significantly. The practice of defensive medicine, which had been a key factor in the cost spiral, seems to have been successfully checked.

Choice and Autonomy

General Discussion

Autonomy is valued by both health caregivers and consumers of health care services. In general, health care professionals will have greater autonomy if they are financially secure and their freedom to conduct their professions is not encumbered with administrative rules and administrators with no health care background. They will have less autonomy if they are dependent on a funding source whose control is at the helm of administrators or bureaucrats without a health care background.

In the health care market, consumers' autonomy is complicated by their lack of information. In the name of protection of consumers, governments often regulate the practice of health caregivers through a licensing system, as a result of which consumers give up the autonomy of consulting certain practitioners whose practice is deemed illegal. One could argue that licensing of doctors, nurses, and other professionals notwithstanding, consumers should be allowed to use the services of unlicensed practitioners at their own risk, as long as these practitioners do not misrepresent their qualifications. On the other hand, one could also argue that the risk is too large, that the benefit is dubious, and that uninformed autonomy is no autonomy at all. There can be no consensus in this debate.

Still, this discussion shows that consumers need the support of independent, medically knowledgeable persons to exercise true autonomy. There is a need for professional patients' advocates.

Consumers will have more autonomy over the quality of services available if they have a role in determining the quality and availability of health care services. Consumers' autonomy in respect to treatment or medical procedures is generally not an issue because consumers do not have expert knowledge of the implications of various treatments and procedures. However, there is agreement that, in the event of a risky operation, they need to be consulted and their consent should be obtained. Further, it is generally regarded as desirable that, as far as possible, consumers should have choice over doctors and over whether or not to seek a second medical opinion in case of doubt.

Like most good things in life, autonomy carries cost. First, autonomy may lead to higher costs because doctors may recommend services and equipment purchases whose benefits may not justify their costs. Second, greater autonomy on the part of consumers will lead to higher administration costs, as well as consumption of services that are too costly to be socially justifiable. Third, autonomy may have moral costs. Society may not, for instance, tolerate abortions, euthanasia, and the selling and buying of organs.

Clearly, society has to consciously make a collective decision in some of these issues; otherwise, the decision may be made by default, and such a decision may be unjustified.

Policy Options

In Hong Kong, producers and consumers of health care services in the private sector enjoy a high degree of autonomy. Their autonomy is circumscribed only by the moral standards of the society and by government regulations. There is nothing the government can do about moral standards in the short run, and there is no scientific basis to judge which moral standards are right or wrong. However, government regulations must be evaluated on the basis of a benefit-cost comparison. If they are found to be worthwhile, then it is important that we learn to live with whatever loss in autonomy those regulations imply.

Within the public sector of Hong Kong's health care system, there is a choice between giving health care professionals autonomy in managing the resources and imposing more regulations. The regulations are generally intended to contain costs, to uphold quality, or for both objectives. They may be in the form of:

1. Budget caps with autonomy over use of funds within the budget;
2. Regulation regarding charges;
3. Required approvals for spending on a case by case basis or for specific categories of spending;
4. Record keeping and disclosure requirements;
5. Licensing requirements; and
6. Setting of standard procedures to provide for accountability.

In principle, budget caps provide health care professionals with a considerable degree of autonomy over the use of resources and the setting of priorities. However, together with regulations regarding charges, consumers are deprived of the autonomy to pay more for better services — unless they opt out of the public hospital system.

As shown in the survey reported in Chapter 2, many households are willing to pay more taxes in return for better public hospital services. There appears clearly a case for setting up some kind of mechanism so that consumers have a part to play in determining the overall quality of health care and how it is to be financed.

The regulatory framework and the judicial system may also affect autonomy. In particular, if the courts are too ready to side with the alleged victims of malpractice and tend to hand out very large indemnities to complainants against malpractice, doctors will have to respond with defensive medicine in an attempt to shift this cost to patients. When this happens, individuals do not have the choice to say, "I am willing to forfeit the right to sue. I am willing to entrust care to a physician I can trust and take the consequences. Give me low-cost care."

An illustration of the cloudiness of the merits of licensing regulations is the fact that while doctors trained in Commonwealth countries were traditionally given the privilege of being allowed to practice in Hong Kong without undergoing a professional examination, all non-Hong Kong-trained doctors are now required to pass such an examination. In the first professional examination after the implementation of the new regulation, as it happened, all candidates from Commonwealth countries failed! One wonders whether all graduates from the two medical schools in Hong Kong would pass the same examination either, and whether the professional examination is just a means to protect the interests of local graduates.

In principle, many of these and similar regulations are intended to protect the interest of patients. One could argue that they are being used to protect the interest of the professionals already practising in Hong Kong. Some regulations, like regulations against abortion and euthanasia, are a means to preserve certain values in a society. Clearly, individual choice, societal values, and group interests may conflict. The actual degree of autonomy of the individuals is often an outcome of conscious or implicit political decision making.

Contrary to common belief, a free market in health care services may not offer the highest degree of free choice and autonomy. With adverse selection being a common market phenomenon, insurance companies have no incentive to offer high-level protection. Individual consumers cannot tell an insurance company, "Even though I am risk averse and want more protection, I am only an average-risk person. Give me a policy that offers me more protection and charge me a fair insurance premium." The problem of adverse selection arises because of high information costs in preventing insurers from distinguishing high-risk clients from low-risk clients. While high information costs make it difficult for an insurance company to distinguish high-cost clients from low-cost ones, sometimes insurance companies are able to tell which groups of individuals are the most costly to insure, for instance, those with chronic illnesses. As a result, these individuals cannot buy insurance. A free market may not give us the freedom or the opportunity to insure against chronic illnesses.

It seems clear from the above discussion that autonomy and choice are likely to be maximized by an appropriate interfacing of the private and the public sectors, and that a formal mechanism of collective decision making will be more satisfactory than decisions made by default or dictated by historical circumstances.

Total Burden and How it is Shared

General Discussion

Total burden refers to the totality of resources committed to health care, including those provided publicly and those provided privately. In general, total burden is not a problem as long as the marginal benefit is equal to or greater than the marginal cost of the burden. The question of whether total burden is too large is therefore really one about efficiency. On the other hand, the question about how total burden is shared is one about distribution.

Spending on health care in the private sector is a result of voluntary exchange between health caregivers and consumers.

Total burden should not be a concern as long as these health case givers and consumers operate in an environment that is conducive to efficiency. Some of the features of this environment have already been addressed in connection with moral hazard, risk management, and choice and autonomy. The subject of total burden in relation to private sector health care spending should only be dealt with indirectly by containing supply-side and demand-side moral hazard, but not directly as a budget to be capped.

Spending on health care in the public sector is a cause of concern because it increases the pressure to raise taxes, but usually there is no mechanism to check the worthiness of the increased health spending.

Policy Options

In order to put a limit to the escalation of public spending on health care, some countries have set global budget caps on tax-funded health care expenditures. The caps may be in the form of a specified percentage of total public expenditures or in the form of a restraint on the percentage increase of revenue appropriated for health care. Among countries that have adopted expenditure ceilings of one sort or another are Denmark, Belgium, Germany, Ireland, Italy, Spain, Portugal, and the United Kingdom. Among these, some caps are not "global". For example, in Germany, health promotion and certain non-hospital services are not constrained. In Denmark, health expenditures by local governments are negotiated. In both Belgium and Germany, different kinds of expenditures are subject to different caps (Abel-Smith and others, 1995, p. 43)

The merit of budget caps for health expenditure is that they can be effective for containing government sector health expenditures, particularly for avoiding a cost explosion, while leaving the private sector to spend more if it so desires. One demerit of such a device is that, unless combined with an enlightened way of spending the budgeted amount to the advantage of the low-income population, there is a risk that the low-income population may not be able to get needed health care services (an access or quantity problem).

Another problem with global budget caps is that quality may be chosen not explicitly but by default. The desire for better quality service may be suppressed unnecessarily.

Actually, some of these problems can be mitigated by combining global budget caps with a cost-recovery system that is biased in favour of the poor. The global budget normally caps only the amount which is to be financed by taxes. Under the least cost principle, part of the financing should also come from fees, and some from insurance premiums. Different financing mechanisms will have different effects both on efficiency and on the distribution of burden. Combining different approaches provides a way of minimizing efficiency loss and a way of allocating the burdens more equitably.

Under the ability to pay principle, those with higher ability to pay should pay more. One could achieve this by offering price discounts to eligible low-income people when they need government-provided health care services. This approach can be described as price-based transfers to the poor. A related approach is discriminatory pricing whereby very low prices would be charged for basic services, but much higher prices for better or superior services. This approach is used in both Singapore and in Hong Kong, and it has the advantage of dispensing with the means test. Self-selection by patients helps allocate the subsidized services to the low income. In a sense, the long queues for government clinics achieve the same purpose. High cost of time for high-income patients effectively drives them away from subsidized services.

Alternatively, one could set different yearly health-related spending limits that vary with different income levels. This approach can be described as *cap*-based transfers to the poor. From the risk-management point of view, the latter approach may be more attractive, as households will know that their health care expenditures will not exceed the stipulated thresholds. In principle there should be a conscious collective choice over the burden–quality combination for publicly provided health care. Other things being equal, raising the burden level by raising the spending thresholds allows the quality of services to be improved.

Conclusions

It may be surprising that a hot topic, cost containment, has not been discussed here explicitly. Containment of spending on health care should never be an issue in and of itself, even though rapid cost escalation does appear to be a problem in many countries. The fact is, increases in spending may be efficient. Focusing on cost containment as such may put emphasis where it does not belong. The important thing is to have the right incentive structure so that efficiency is achieved. It is important then to accept whatever spending level occurs under these conditions.

Expensive technology would thus be worthwhile if the benefits are larger than the costs. Investing in medical research would be worthwhile if the expected benefits outweigh the costs. Skill development would be worthwhile if it yields net benefit and not worthwhile if it does not.

Moral hazard is a real problem in the health care market, and it certainly has much to do with cost. Moral hazard is especially serious when risks are underwritten by a third party — particularly if underwritten by the government — and when the claims are made by health care providers who profit from the claims. However, the challenge lies in designing risk-management systems that can provide the right incentives, and not in containing costs as such.

There are peculiarities in the medical care market that present difficult problems, and they must be dealt with. These peculiarities have largely to do with information cost. The challenge of designing a sound health care system lies essentially in coming to terms with the principal–agent problem, which is predicated on information cost. Cost containment in neglect of the needs and rising aspirations of the community is inefficient. On the other hand, once there is a system that can provide the right incentives to the different players in the health care equation, waste can be avoided, and efficiency in health care can be achieved. An administratively determined budget cap on health care spending that is unresponsive to consumer demand will not be warranted.

The next chapter will draw on the insight gained from the analysis thus far in order to offer recommendations which will provide the basis for a healthier health-care system.

Notes

1. The U.S. Tax Equity and Fiscal Reform Act of 1982 created 470 Diagnostic Related Groups after an experimental plan in New Jersey (Morreim 1995, p. 15). In Hong Kong the Hospital Authority uses the term Patient-Related Group (PRG).

2. *Ming Pao* (31 October 1996) had a story about an incident in a private hospital. A senior surgeon associated with a private hospital proposed to do an appendectomy on a case that he alleged to be one of appendicitis when, in actual fact, it was nothing of the sort. He was only prevented from doing the surgery when a colleague and friend of the patient's mother intervened.

CHAPTER 5

Recommendations

Introduction

We need a health care system that can do the following:

1. Protect people from the risk of unexpectedly large health care expenditure;
2. Resolve the principal–agent problem[1] so that health care professionals' interest corresponds with patients' interest;
3. Provide access to quality basic care for all members of society while allowing the choice for better care, including state-of-the-art care, for those who opt for it;
4. Maintain sufficient incentives for households to engage in a healthy lifestyle and in preventive activities; and
5. Provide a mechanism whereby a collective, intelligent decision can be made regarding the trade-off between quality and burden.

We put forward four sets of recommendations in this chapter as an effort in meeting such a need. In a nutshell, we recommend that a universal health insurance plan be implemented in tandem with private health insurance; that providers of health care in the private sector be allowed to have more freedom in (re-)organizing themselves to work more efficiently with health providers in the public sector; that cost and budget caps be applied and malpractice compensations be awarded with consideration of their effects on the health care system; and that professional autonomy and freedom of choice be upheld by adopting schemes from abroad that would effectively check unnecessary intrusions. These are explained in order.

A Universal Excess Burden Health Insurance Plan (UEBHIP)

Universal Insurance for All

Without intervention or assistance from the government, private insurers generally do not want to insure known chronic patients. Private insurers may not insure certain groups of people regarded as being in high risk groups. To the extent that every member of society needs protection from the risk of large health care expenditures due to long-term health problems or unexpected illnesses, a risk-pooling mechanism that provides universal coverage is recommended.

A mandatory savings plan for health care expenditures is not recommended because each individual will have to give up a lot of consumption for a long time in order to have a reasonable degree of protection. The popularity of Medishield in Singapore, which is optional on top of the mandatory Medisave, shows that a mandatory savings plan is inadequate.

The main merit of a mandatory savings plan for health care is said to be its ability to contain demand-side moral hazard (see Chapter 4). This objective, however, can be more effectively and more efficiently achieved by making households responsible for their health care expenditures up to a yearly threshold. This recommended approach is more effective than a scheme like Medisave because a Medisave plan may not do much to contain demand-side moral hazard; it is especially so if the Medisave account has no alternative use apart from health care spending. It is more efficient also because mandated savings cannot possibly accommodate the different needs and preferences of different households. In contrast, if households are responsible for their own health care expenditures (up to a yearly threshold), those that adopt a healthier lifestyle as well as those that start off with a better health status (better genes, for example) may rationally choose to save less for their medical needs.

A risk-pooling mechanism that provides insurance against excessive health care spending need not be financed by the collection of risk-differentiated premiums. Indeed, the collection of risk-differentiated premiums would run counter to an important objective of health policy, namely, accessibility to quality basic care. As argued in Chapter 2, a key feature of the health care system in Hong Kong today is a universal basic health insurance plan that is tax financed.

The distinguishing characteristic of an insurance plan is that members contribute to a pool and draw from it in the event that the insured contingency occurs. Hong Kong residents contribute into the public sector health care budget by paying taxes, and enjoy the protection that is made possible by the resources thus made available. Of course some Hong Kong residents do not pay taxes, and some pay very little. The assumption might be made that they had received transfers from the government and had paid from the transfers. Alternatively, the assumption might be that their contribution had been subsidized by others.

The best scheme would involve the continuation of a tax-financed universal basic health insurance plan (the Basic Plan) which would be modified to become a Universal Excess Burden Health Insurance Plan (UEBHIP). A portion of the financing of UEBHIP would come from user charges.

User Charges

The Basic Plan would require a household to register the number of household members covered. The household will pay all direct costs for the use of covered health care services by its members, up to a yearly limit based on the number of members in the household. The distinction between direct costs and overhead costs is delineated in Appendix B.

For administrative simplicity, it is proposed that this yearly spending limit be set at a uniform per capita rate basis rather than varying with income or the number of members in the household,

Table 5.1

Yearly Health Spending Limits for a Typical Hong Kong Household (3.3 members)* (illustrative only, dollars are at 1996 prices)

Net Income after Tax / Transfer	Yearly Health Spending Limit (threshold)
Public assistance recipients	0
Household income below 1.5 x median income (on application)	3%** of yearly median household income (=HK$ 6,300)
All others	6% of yearly median household income (=HK$ 12,600)

Notes: * Numbers are for illustrative purposes only. Actual numbers must be socially determined; 3.3 is the average household size in the 1996 By-census; median monthly income is HK$17,500.

** In the consultation document "Towards Better Health", based on the average hospital stay of 4.4 days per patient in HA hospitals, it was stated that the proposed hospital charges amounted to only 2.8% of median household income and was therefore acceptable. That proposed formula ignored cases where the hospital stay was longer or where household income was smaller than the median. Our formula ensures that yearly spending on health care need not exceed the stated percentages unless the household voluntarily opts for better quality at higher cost.

(although the latter is theoretically preferred). There are rooms for adjustment. The household spending limit should be zero for those falling below the poverty line, and the limit may be reduced for households meeting certain eligibility criteria (Table 5.1).

User charges should be arrived at after detailed analysis of the fixed cost, variable cost and especially the marginal cost. Appendix B shows how to divide up, in practice, the total cost into these three types of costs. Here marginal costs refer to the direct costs arising from the use of health care services, such as drugs, materials, laboratory tests, food and accommodation, service-related capital-depreciation charges, and a percentage of manpower costs attributable to patient care. For two reasons, payments for manpower costs should not be relied upon to cover the entire cost of hiring the medical staff: (1) the medical staff have other duties not directly related to patient care, and (2) doctors provide valuable standby service even when they are not seeing patients. As a matter of principle, payments should not attempt to cover any part of fixed costs which do not vary with patient care. The latter should be financed by taxes.

To make the scheme viable, four overriding principles should be closely observed. The first principle is that households should be responsible for their health care expenditures if demand-side moral hazard is to be checked. Holding households responsible for health care charges within the spending limit will encourage them to adopt a healthier lifestyle. The second is that households must not be exposed to excessive risks. Shielding households from expenditures beyond the spending limit will provide the necessary assurance. The third is that charges should stay close to marginal costs in order to control supply-side moral hazard. The proposed setup should remove the incentive to oversupply services. Finally, overhead costs for health care, personnel costs included, should be incurred on the basis of a social benefit-cost analysis. Spending on the basis of comparing social benefit and social cost is more efficient than arbitrary budget caps.

In short, the proposed system draws on the general tax revenue to pay for expenditures on eligible services over the stipulated spending limits for households, and to pay for all overhead expenditures related to health care. Households whose incomes fall below the poverty line may be subject to lower charges or be exempt from charges altogether.[2] Alternatively, households may still be required to pay the direct-cost charges while being given a transfer in the form of a yearly health budget. The latter approach is in principle more efficient if the poor households truly believe that the government will not come to their assistance when they run out of cash. Otherwise, the poor households may use the extra transfer to boost their non-health-related spending and bet that the government would bail them out when they could not come up with the resources to pay for health care.

Choice for Better Services

Under the proposed scheme, households have the option to spend more to get more than the standard, covered services. If they do so, the extra spending would not count towards the spending limit. After breaching the spending limit, standard services will all be covered by the government, but households may get better services, if they so desire, by supplementing government-paid charges with extra spending from their own pockets.

It is proposed that the Hospital Authority (HA) enter into contracts with private hospitals so that patients can be referred to them, with standard fees for standard services being chargeable to the patient if the yearly spending limit has not been reached, and be chargeable to the government if the yearly spending limit has been exceeded. In principle, the contracts would involve the Hospital Authority giving the private hospitals a lump sum payment at the beginning of the year, thus contributing towards their overhead expenditures. The private hospitals will then be committed to charging fees that cover direct costs when they look after patients referred from HA hospitals. Again, patients may choose to opt for better than standard services by paying more.

Allowing HA doctors to refer patients to private hospitals, or letting patients to opt for care in private hospitals, will relieve HA hospitals of their excessive patient load and thus improve the quality of services. Since many private hospitals are presently facing a problem of underutilization of facilities, the proposed arrangement should help improve the financial positions of these private hospitals.

Administrative Problems

Because all eligible health care expenditures are chargeable to the household's account regardless of whether its members consult a private doctor or a government clinic, the UEBHIP scheme requires that a central file be set up for each household. It may be noted that the patient will have much incentive to ensure that all eligible health care payments are recorded in the central files. The setup provides a self-monitoring mechanism for accurate filing of doctors' incomes.

The advent of modern computer technology has made the maintenance of a central file easier than before. The operation of the scheme requires: the recording of patients' payments for standard services; billing by authorized caregivers for services rendered in excess of household spending limits and paying the caregivers by the government; and periodic auditing of the honesty of the caregivers and patients.

A possible question about the operation of the proposed scheme is whether households, realizing that excess payments will be covered by the government, might speed up their utilization of the health care system. This scenario, however, is unlikely to arise because having to use the services of the health care system is not an enjoyable experience. In particular, exhausting the spending limit quickly boils down to spending more money from the household's own pocket. More importantly, even though a household has not spent up to the spending limit, the government still stands ready to assist as soon as the spending limit is exceeded. There is really no advantage to quickly breaching the spending limit.

Better Quality than Currently Possible

Compared to the current system, the government will amass extra resources through charges, and such resources that can be utilized to support an improvement in the quality of health care. In particular, the length of the queues can be reduced.

However, the plan will have to pay standard charges to private health care agents when a household's spending limit has been exceeded. If the health care agent charges in excess of the standard charges, the household is responsible for paying the excess. There is some risk that private hospitals may over-supply services at the expense of taxpayers if patients pay extra charges. But this is not expected to be a major concern. Overall, the government will have more resources for medical care.

Private Health Insurance

The proposed UEBHIP scheme leaves a lot of room for private health insurance to play important roles. First, private insurance may offer protection from the standard charges (marginal cost charges) for which households are responsible before the spending limit has been reached. Second, private insurance may cover excess charges when better-than-standard services are rendered such as better accommodation (semi-private or private rooms) when a patient is hospitalized. Third, private insurance may pay for extra, state-of-the-art care that is not included in the Basic Plan.

When a patient is covered in the private plan, all standard charges paid by the insurance company on behalf of the patient, up to the spending limit, should still be centrally recorded, so that the patient will enjoy the exemption from standard charges after the spending limit has been reached.

The existence of spending limits, beyond which the government will cover marginal cost, will help contain private health insurance cost for citizens. The private plans may or may not require co-payment or deductible charges. Thus there will be a large range of choices available, catering to varying needs of households for risk containment.

The Role of Private Health Care Providers

Doctors in private practice can take patients with or without referral from government doctors. They have to keep a record of their patients' medical history and treatment and to file records of charges to the UEBHIP scheme. Prior to reaching the yearly spending limits, they can charge whatever they like as long as the patients consent to paying for the charges (although only standard charges can count towards the account). After the yearly spending thresholds have been breached, the Plan will start paying for the charges at the stipulated rates set by the government or the Hospital Authority. Patients may, however, top up the charges with extra payments if this is agreeable to them. Health care providers should let their patients know what rates they charge. In principle, doctors and hospitals agreeing to abide by the rates set by the government (via HA) will receive an annual prospective payment to help cover their overhead costs.

Private hospitals can admit patients of their own accord, or admit patients referred by government doctors. To the extent that, under the proposed arrangement, HA hospitals will charge patients marginal costs rather than nominal fees (as they do now) prior to their reaching the yearly spending limits, private hospitals will be in a much better position to compete with HA hospitals for patients. Further, to the extent that private hospitals receive prospective payments in addition to fees, they will also have more room for survival.

Private practices should, under the Plan, be free to organize themselves as Health Maintenance Organizations (HMOs). Members of the public who subscribe to an HMO will pay all necessary fees which are counted as "contingent credit" (to be explained below) towards the yearly spending limit. If annual charges exceed the threshold, however, the government will not pay the excess because the subscribers are assumed to be getting more than the basic protection under the universal plan. When members of HMOs actually use the health care services supplied by their HMOs, the imputed standard charges will validate dollar for dollar the contingent credit already recorded. After imputed charges have exceeded the spending limits, the government will start paying the standard charges to the HMO. In general, this provision of the Plan will be reflected in the form of lower subscription fees for HMO members. The government must not pay the patient because that would induce demand. As the fees paid to the HMOs cover only marginal cost, supply-side moral hazard should not be a problem. The HMO model offers an extra choice to households. Those HMOs that are efficient and innovative can attract members by offering superior services while containing costs. In any case, if HMOs can survive the market test, they can be said to have served a useful purpose.

Tax-paid Doctors as Patient Advocates

Consumers of health care services are generally not in the position to judge the quality of health care services provided by private medical service providers. Following the proposal made by Maynard in Chapter 4, it is proposed that the government finance a number of clinics which are manned by tax-paid, salaried doctors. These doctors may provide consultation services and may refer patients to other doctors and hospitals. When they provide referral services, they will serve as patients' advocates. In case of need, and with the consent of patients, government doctors acting as patients' advocates can access the medical history of patients kept by private practitioners.

The reason such tax-paid doctors would serve well as patients' advocates is that they have no financial interest in the treatment of the patient. As professionals whose income is not related to the number of patient visitations, they are in a good position to command the trust of patients. However, it does not follow that patients will only visit government-operated facilities. The availability of government doctors to serve as advocates only provides an additional option for patients who need extra advice and who need an informed second opinion about costly services and procedures recommended by private practitioners.

Cost Containment, Global Budget Caps, and Malpractice Compensation

Will the system described above contribute toward cost containment? Will there be a role for a cap for tax-financed expenditures on health care? This section will attempt to answer these questions. Under the system described above, the revenue for financing health care expenditures in the entire economy is derived from several sources:

1. Tax revenue, which finances health infrastructure acquisition and maintenance, and excess household spending on health services over the spending limits;
2. Standard fees and charges paid by households, before their yearly spending limits have been reached to finance the

variable costs of standard health care services in both private and public sector services;

3. Extra payments for non-standard services;
4. Health insurance payments to cover pre-spending-limit standard charges and to provide extra services; and
5. HMO subscription fees paid by households or employers.

Of all these items, only part of the first item can and should be capped. Tax-financed health infrastructure expenditures should be capped in order to prevent impulsive or unwarranted purchases. Modern health equipment is extremely expensive and should be carefully evaluated in terms of cost and benefit before being acquired. Nevertheless, the caps should not be rigid in that when a carefully conducted cost-benefit analysis justifies a purchase, the cap should be relaxed to accommodate it.

Clearly, if the government finds its spending over the household annual thresholds too onerous — that it has to cut back other areas of spending or to limit excessively the quality of health care services — it can increase the annual spending limit and thus increase the burden borne by citizens. Raising the annual spending limit need not adversely affect accessibility if a lower limit (even zero) may apply to the poor. Alternatively, in the face of excessive burden, the government can lower the quality of standard services to be provided. This again highlights the perennial three-way trade-off among burden, accessibility, and quality. It is highly desirable that to have a formal mechanism for collective decision-making about the quality of health care services desired — given the quality-burden trade-off and assuming that accessibility and efficiency are immutable or have already been achieved.

One additional observation is that the explosion of health care expenditures in the United States has been caused by the prevalence of malpractice suits that end up with large awards. Such awards have led to high malpractice insurance premiums which are then passed on to patients. Another consequence has been the rise of the practice of defensive medicine. Defensive medicine refers to the practice of prescribing normally unwarranted procedures or diagnostic tests in order to avoid even the slightest chance of being sued for malpractice. The experience of the United States clearly indicates that awards for malpractice compensation should be given with a broader perspective in regard to implications for the cost of health care. Unwarranted, large malpractice awards may have a perverse effect on the quality of health care because, by increasing burden unnecessarily, either quality or accessibility would have to be sacrificed. Resources would be diverted to pay for the cost of malpractice insurance premiums and litigation at the expense of proper health care.

Autonomy and Freedom of Choice

Autonomy, in the sense of respect for professionalism and freedom from bureaucratic interference, is very important for lifting morale among medical professionals and for improving the quality of medical services. This autonomy is, however, sometimes compromised on budgetary grounds. Once the supply-side and demand-side moral hazards are contained — through setting charges on the basis of marginal cost and through the limited household responsibility arrangements — overspending that prompts budget cuts will be less of a problem. Administrative rules that reduce professional autonomy will then be unnecessary.

The Canadian experience demonstrates clearly how budgetary considerations have eroded autonomy and undermined morale in the health care profession. To control runaway costs resulting from excessive billing under a system of third-party insurance by the government, the Province of Ontario in Canada has passed a law, under the name of the Savings and Restructuring Act, that has empowered the Minister of Health to unilaterally close hospitals, announce regions where doctors are oversupplied and therefore no longer welcome, and to rescind payment for services that government inspectors found unnecessary (Arnett, Jr. 1996). The law came into effect in January 1996.

Apart from these intrusions into professional practice, the Ontario government has also introduced an intricate, progressive "clawback" mechanism to keep a lid on ballooning health care costs. Doctors are required to return to the government one-third of their gross yearly income over C$251,000, two-thirds of incomes over C$276,000, and three-fourths of incomes over C$301,000. According to Arnett, doctors are leaving Ontario in large numbers, to the extent that 30 of the 95 family medicine graduates at a Canadian university had left for the U.S. in 1995, while 80 among 95 of the 1996 graduates indicated a desire to emigrate. The Ontario experience suggests that private provision of medical services is not a sufficient condition for autonomy.

It is clear from comparing with the Canadian model that the current system in Hong Kong, which is based on salaries as the form of remuneration to public sector medical practitioners, does provide a good basis for achieving professional autonomy. Since the economic gains of doctors are not related to the service provided, there is no need to worry about them oversupplying consultation services. There is, however, still concern that doctors may prescribe tests and drugs without being fully aware of whether the tests and drugs are cost effective. With allocation of budgets based on expected spending which, in the case of nine major acute hospitals in Hong Kong, are partly based on the number of patients expected to be admitted in each Patient-Related Group (PRG)[3], doctors can be trusted to exercise their autonomy with an awareness of cost. It should be noted that in Hong Kong the annual budgets allocated to hospitals are rigidly adhered to.[4] It is up to each hospital to think of innovative and cost-effective ways to deliver their services most cost effectively.

Still, this autonomy will increase if hospitals have access to a larger source of revenue than currently available. The "payment subject to the spending limit" arrangement proposed herein will help procure an additional source of revenue, thus contributing to an increase in autonomy.

On the demand side, consumers will have the following autonomy: over the kind of insurance that they want to buy for protection against spending within the spending limits, or for better-than-standard services; and autonomy over the combination of burden and quality of public sector health care services available. This second autonomy is to be achieved through a collective decision mechanism that takes into account the trade-off between burden and quality. The government, through the Hospital Authority, should provide information about this trade-off so consumers can make an intelligent decision. The choice is to be made simply by setting the annual spending threshold. A higher spending threshold implies greater burden and, assuming efficiency is maintained, higher quality.

Conclusions

Aaron (1994, pp. 31–32) submits that the goals of health care reform are well known: to assure citizens of a country financial access to health care, to slow the growth of health care spending, and to sustain or improve the quality of care. He does not believe that voluntary actions of businesses and individuals will achieve the first goal. Some form of mandate, either on individuals or on businesses, or some form of direct government provision, is necessary.

The best approach to ensuring financial accessibility is to set a household-level annual spending threshold beyond which the government would step in and take over the burden. It will be up to the individual households, or the employers of the breadwinners of households, to buy additional insurance for them. The additional insurance may protect them from payment within the threshold or avail them of better-than-basic health care. So long as the thresholds are set at levels that are compatible with financial accessibility, there will be no need for a mandate.

The best approach to contain health care spending is to structure incentives efficiently. Making households responsible for within-threshold health care spending will induce more prevention and a healthier lifestyle. Reducing the financial incentive to supply services by setting charges at the level of direct costs, while providing prospective payments to pay for overheads, will ensure efficient delivery of health care services.

Providing quality care is a non-issue. The crucial question is about what quality is preferred, given the trade-off between quality and burden. Provided that the delivery of health care services is efficient, and assuming that a consensus over accessibility has been reached, the next important question is how to establish optimal quality on the basis of consumer preference. The array of health care services that are to be provided subject to government subsidy must be expressly determined. It is necessary to have a mechanism that can relate the trade-off between quality and burden to consumers. It is also necessary to have a mechanism for households to choose the quality-burden combination that they want. This is an aspect of consumers' sovereignty. We have argued and concluded that the proposed universal insurance plan (UEBHIP) would best balance the various trade-offs and lead to viable, high-quality system of health care in Hong Kong.

Notes

1. See Chapter 4, section on "Moral Hazard (Producers Side)" problems. When the principal–agent problem is solved, health care professionals will want to improve the health of the patients while minimizing costs, and will want to acquire new skills or refresh old skills that are beneficial to the patients.

2. We are aware that ascertaining the poverty line and the eligibility criteria would complicate the administration of the proposed scheme.

3. According to a document of the Finance Committee of the Hospital Authority under the title "Application of Specialty and PRG Costing to 1996 / 97 Resource Allocation", "the 1996 / 97 resource allocation formula for the nine major acute hospitals calls for 30% of these hospitals' budgets to be allocated based on the average costs of patient output of each clinical specialty adjusted for 'case mix' by PRGs." (p. 2)

4. This is unlike the French case. Notwithstanding caps dating from the early 1970s under the name *taux directeur*, exceptions or "derogations" were allowed. Hospitals could spend above the caps if the unplanned expenses were justified. As a result of this, greater autonomy was achieved at the expense of routine overspending (see Mosse 1994).

CHAPTER 6

Epilogue

Alternative Viable Models: the Singapore Model and Hay's Model

The Singapore Model and the ChoiceCare Model (proposed by Hay in 1992) are viable alternatives to the present HA system, but each has some serious drawbacks. In the Epilogue, we intend to show that our preferred model, the UEBHIP model, has worked well in another country.

Both the Singapore Model and Hay's ChoiceCare Model give much greater role to the private sector than the HA system now as implemented. The central element of the Singapore Model is the Medisave Plan, a forced savings plan tied to the Central Provident Fund Scheme. The Medisave Plan was introduced in 1984. In essence, funds are accumulated to be spent on health care when need arises. The health system in Singapore has been improved recently to provide catastrophe insurance through a new Medishield scheme (implemented in 1990) and redistributive assistance to the poor through the Medifund (implemented in 1993). As Table 6.1 shows, the Medisave Plan appears very effective in decreasing the burden on the public purse of providing for health care.

The main problem with the Singapore system is that the funds accumulated may be inadequate for some households and too large for others. When they have become too large, there is a good likelihood that they will be expended in a socially suboptimal way. The fact that the mandatory savings in the Medisave Plan can only be used for approved medical expenditures means that they do not

Table 6.1

Impact of the Medisave Plan of Singapore, 1982–94

Types of Hospitals	1982	1994
% of patients admitted to private hospitals and Class A wards in public hospitals	17	32
% of patients admitted to heavily subsidized Class C wards in public hospitals	66	19

Source: Kwa (1996).

Notes: Charges for Class A wards are based on full-cost pricing.

have an opportunity cost to their owners. As such, they tend to be overexpended. There is even a possibility that households that have accumulated a large pool of money in their Medisave accounts may take less preventive actions to avoid health hazards. Naturally the private health care sector stands to gain from such an arrangement, and the government's fiscal burden is lightened. But it may not be efficient from society's point of view. To an extent, this problem has now been alleviated by a provision allowing households to stop contributions when their Medisave accounts have reached a certain level.

The essence of Hay's ChoiceCare Plan lies in allowing individuals greater choice over the disposition of the per capita public funds that are set aside notionally for each citizen by the government. The individual can opt to take out this money to pay in whole or in part for any of the private plans offered in the marketplace as well as plans sponsored by local HA hospitals. Alternatively, the individual can choose none of these plans and stay in the existing health care system.

The Plan may be viable in a modified form but not viable as it currently stands. The main problem is that average cost is distinct from marginal cost. Given all the infrastructure already available, the opting out of any individual from the existing health care system will increase the average cost of health care for the remaining citizens. As an individual opts out from the public system, he (she) takes the average cost budget with him (her) to the private plan but saves only the marginal cost of health care for the public system. This in itself would pose a serious financial strain on the public system; but there is another problem. Those who opt out of the public system are likely to be healthier individuals who are welcome by the private sector rather than individuals with chronic health problems. Although Hay would like to impose a condition on all private plans that they must not discriminate against anyone on the basis of age or pre-existing health conditions, the public may perceive an enforcement problem. As a result, the chronically sick or those who are vulnerable to long-term health problems are likely to stay inside the public system, which would inevitably run into difficulty maintaining quality without an infusion of more public funds.

If Hay's Plan is to work, those who decide to opt out must not take the average cost budget with them but only an amount equal to the expected marginal cost of servicing them. This is likely to be much smaller than the average cost budget. But if they take away anything more than the expected marginal cost of servicing them within the public system, the average cost for the remaining citizens will definitely rise.

Despite these practical difficulties, the spirit of Hay's Choice-Care Plan is commendable. Citizens should have greater choice over the quality of health care. They should have the freedom to pay more for better services. The private sector should have a greater role to play, both in terms of underwriting health insurance policies and in terms of supplying health care services. The Universal Excess Burden Health Insurance Plan (UEBHIP) allows the private sector to play both roles. (see p. 84)

The Workability of UEBHIP

The proposal made in this book, namely, the Universal Excess Burden Health Insurance Plan, actually is alive and working in Sweden. According to OECD (1994), in Sweden "the patient's combined cost for medical treatment and drugs is restricted to a maximum of

Skr. 1,600 per annum, after which further treatment and drugs are free of charge" (p. 271). The Swedish national government allocates funds to county councils and three municipalities which administer medical care services for their populations. The greater majority of medical professionals are employees of the counties or municipalities who draw salaries from the authorities, even though, under an experimental system, some of them now derive a compensation related to the services they provide. About 8% of all physicians in Sweden engage in private practice. Yet many of them have agreements with county councils and receive compensation from them according to a prespecified formula when they deliver services to patients. This is almost exactly the scheme proposed here for Hong Kong.

Under the Swedish system, a patient who visits the County Health Centre, the Accident and Emergency Departments of hospitals, or who is admitted as an inpatient of county hospitals, pays standard fees set by the county for the services he or she obtains. But his (her) total approved health care expenditures are limited to a ceiling set by the national government. It is interesting to note that, despite this underwriting by the government for all recognized health care spending above the yearly spending limit, Sweden contains its health-care expenditures exceedingly well. Indeed, Sweden is a unique country in that health-care expenditures as a percentage of the GDP actually *fell* noticeably in the 1980s, from 9.4% to 8.6%. The degree of decline is even more impressive when we note that the share of public expenditures on health care in the GDP fell from 8.7% to 7.8%.

Advertising and the Future of the Health Care Market

In Hong Kong, advertising by doctors is not allowed according to the code of professional ethics maintained by the Hong Kong Medical Council. Doctors can only advertise the opening or the moving of their clinics but they cannot advertise their fees or their expertise. This practice is damaging to effective competition.

Although it makes sense in the interest of the public to outlaw unsubstantiated claims, there is little justification for the banning of factual advertising. The banning of medical factual advertising can only be construed as motivated by the self-interest of the profession against erosion of profits by competition.

Under the Plan, as explained above, there is scope for partnership between the private practitioners and the public sector doctors. Hong Kong belongers who are covered by the Plan may see a private doctor as they please, but only the standard charges against recognized services would count towards the yearly spending limit and would be paid with public money once the spending limit has been exceeded. It is therefore very important that patients know how much doctors are charging for what services.

A Medical Ombudsman for Hong Kong?

In Sweden, complaints from patients against doctors or nurses are handled by the National Board of Health and Welfare, although they may also be directed to the Medical Disciplinary Board. If a complaint is substantiated, the case is referred to the Medical Disciplinary Board, which may withdraw or limit the right of a physician or a nurse to practice in his or her profession. Every year the Board administers about 300 admonitions and warnings, and withdraws 10 to 15 work authorizations from physicians, dentists, and nurses. These figures are quite large given that Sweden has a population of 8.6 million. In Hong Kong, complaints from patients against medical professionals are lodged with the Hong Kong Medical Council, which received a total of 168 complaints against doctors in 1996 — a somewhat lower figure compared to the 177 complaints in 1995 and 170 complaints in 1994. Currently, these complaints are investigated by professionals who are very often themselves in private practice. This is not desirable. In general, investigators should be full-time, salaried professionals who do nothing but act as independent investigators. It is highly desirable that the results of investigations are available for the public to review so that consumers of medical services can look at the record of their doctors.

Table 6.2

Fees of Primary Care Services Supplied by Department of Health, HA Hospitals

Service	Fee (from 15 November 1996)
General outpatient consultation	$37*
Specialist outpatient consultation (dermatology)	$44
Dressing / injection only	$15
Families clinic	$ 1
Social hygiene clinic (venereal diseases)	Free
Tuberculosis and chest clinic	Free

Source: Department of Health, Hospital Authority.
Note: *$195 for non-Hong Kong belongers.

Conclusions

On the whole, Hong Kong has a sound health care system. The government, through either the Hospital Authority system of hospitals or the Department of Health clinics, runs a heavily subsidized primary care service (Table 6.2). No means test is required. But the services, in particular outpatient services are almost exclusively used by the low and middle-income population through a mechanism of self-selection. Higher income individuals generally opt for private sector health service because high value of their time makes it uneconomical for them to spend time waiting in queues. An ambulatory service, open 24 hours a day and available in a number of HA hospitals, provides emergency service to patients in need in order of urgency or seriousness of the health problem.

The waiting time for attending government clinics is generally felt to be long and is a sore point emphasized by Joel Hay (1992).

> "The primary cost for many Hong Kong patients visiting government facilities is not monetary, but rather the lost waiting time. This is the main reason why outpatient visits to private doctors outnumber government outpatient clinic visits by nearly 4:1" (p. 22).

What Hay says is quite true. However, assuming that subsidized services should be reserved for the lower income people, it may be argued that an administrative machinery to conduct a means test to determine eligibility may be more costly than relying on queues and self-selection to ration services.

The Hong Kong health system is laudable in terms of financial accessibility but not necessarily in terms of physical accessibility. Because of resource constraints, laboratory service is usually not available around the clock, and the heavy demand for services contributes to a delay in diagnosis which can sometimes be fatal. Surgeries are routinely delayed. Patients are often discharged prematurely and admission criteria are tightening up. Improvement of physical accessibility requires a greater commitment of resources, but this must not imply imposing an excessive burden on anyone. Still, no one should be surprised by an unexpectedly large medical bill. The importance of this is being increasingly recognized around the world and is a driving force behind health care reform both in the U.S. and in Europe (McPhee 1995, Abel-Smith et al. 1995).

APPENDIX A

Notes on Three Surveys

Time and Response Rates

The three surveys described here are the Doctors' Survey, the Hospital Administers' Survey, and the Public Survey, all carried out around the end of 1996.

For the Public Survey, 3,936 telephone numbers randomly selected from the residential telephone directory were dialled during the evenings of 19–21 November 1996. The response rate was 29.6%. This is calculated as a percentage out of the total of (a) number of completed interviews and (b) number of eligible households contacted, with or without the target respondent being available. It should be noted that respondents were not prompted verbally for answers even though alternative answers appear on the questionnaires. Respondents could not see the range of answers on the questionnaires, which were provided only for the convenience of the interviewers making the calls.

Hospital Authority (HA) doctors were surveyed with the co-operation of the Hospital Authority Headquarters Office which dispatched the questionnaires together with the Hospital Administrator Questionnaires to the Hospital Chief Executives of each HA hospital. Some questionnaires were returned in bulk; others were returned by mail or by fax. A total of 189 HA doctors were successfully surveyed. The response rate cannot be calculated because Hospital Chief Executives (HEC) were relied on to distribute the questionnaires, and not all HCEs co-operated.

Non-HA doctors were surveyed through questionnaires mailed to all doctors listed in the yellow pages of the telephone directory with full addresses referenced from the Gazette. A total of 61 doctors responded among 248, representing a response rate of 24.6%.

Among public hospitals, 13 Hospital Chief Executives out of a total of 42 participated in the survey. Among 14 private hospitals, 3 responded.

Doctors' Survey, Hong Kong, November 1996

Questionnaires to Doctors

The Hong Kong Centre for Economic Research and Lingnan College of Hong Kong are supporting a study on Hong Kong's medical care system. The study will provide input for the Special Administrative Region government to improve our medical care system. We very much hope that you will assist us by returning the questionnaire below.

Please fax this to: Dr Raymond Ng (2591-0690) or, if you prefer, mail to: Centre for Public Policy Studies, Lingnan College, Tuen Mun, by 15 December 1996. Please direct questions (if any) to: Dr Ho Lok Sang (2616-7178)

All information will be kept strictly confidential. Please *Circle* your answers.

1. Which of the following best describes your current practice?

    a) private practice without affiliation with any private hospital

    b) private practice with affiliation with a private hospital

    c) practice in an HA hospital

    d) practice as an employee of a private hospital

    e) practice as an employee of a company/organization

    f) practice as an employee in nonclinical duties within the public sector

    g) practice as an employee in nonclinical duties in the private sector

2. Please indicate total number of years of clinical practice in your career:

   a) Public sector, Hong Kong _____

   b) Public sector, outside Hong Kong _____

   c) Private sector, Hong Kong _____

   d) Private sector, outside Hong Kong _____

3. How many hours of work per week do you average?

   a) Below 40 hours

   b) 40 to 49 hours

   c) 50 to 59 hours

   d) 60 to 70 hours

   e) Over 70 hours

4. What percentage of your work hours is devoted to clinical duties?
   _____%

5. How do you assess the overall pay package in HA relative to what you can get in private practice?

1	2	3	4	5
Inferior				Superior

6. Do you agree with the following statements?

   a) experience in an HA hospital is useful to career building in the medical profession.

1	2	3	4	5
No				Yes

   b) work in an HA hospital is rewarding as an ultimate career in the medical profession.

1	2	3	4	5
No				Yes

7a. How would you rate professional autonomy in Hong Kong's hospitals?

   HA Hospitals
Low	1	2	3	4	5	High

   Private Hospitals
Low	1	2	3	4	5	High

7b. Do you think the workload in Hong Kong's hospitals is too heavy?

HA Hospitals
No   1   2   3   4   5   Yes
Private Hospitals
No   1   2   3   4   5   Yes

7c. If you indicated that the workload is too heavy, do you think the workload has jeopardized the quality of care?

HA Hospitals
No   1   2   3   4   5   Yes
Private Hospitals
No   1   2   3   4   5   Yes

7d. How much do you agree or disagree with the following statements:

(1 = Very much disagree); (5 = Very much agree)

a) The number of nurses in Hong Kong's hospitals is adequate.

1   2   3   4   5   HA Hospitals
1   2   3   4   5   Private Hospitals

b) Patients receive reasonably good care in Hong Kong's hospitals.

1   2   3   4   5   HA Hospitals
1   2   3   4   5   Private Hospitals

c) Patients in Hong Kong's hospitals are seldom denied the most appropriate care because of a lack of resources.

1   2   3   4   5   HA Hospitals
1   2   3   4   5   Private Hospitals

d) HA hospitals provide generally better quality service to patients than private hospitals.

1   2   3   4   5

e) HA doctors are generally better motivated than private practice doctors to act in the best interest of patients.

1   2   3   4   5

f) Private practice doctors are less handicapped by resource considerations to act in the best interest of patients.

1   2   3   4   5

8. (for those in private practice only) What is the average fee charged for each consultation, including the cost of medication?

_____ dollars

Hospital Administrators' Survey

The Hong Kong Centre for Economic Research and Lingnan College of Hong Kong are supporting a study on Hong Kong's medical care system. The study will provide input for the Special Administrative Region government to improve our medical care system. We very much hope that you will assist us by returning the questionnaire below.

Please fax this to: Dr Raymond Ng (2591-0690) or, if you prefer, Mail to: Centre for Public Policy Studies, Lingnan College, Tuen Mun, by 15 December 1996. Please Direct questions (if any) to: Dr. Ho Lok Sang (2616-7178)

All information will be kept strictly confidential. Please *Circle* your answers.

1. Type:

   a) HA

   b) Non-HA, registered charitable organization

   c) Non-HA, not a registered charitable organization

2. Number of hospital beds _____

3. Percentage of hospital beds utilized on average _____

4. Scale of operation:

   a) Number of full-time staff doctors: _____

   b) Number of full-time nonmedical professional staff (excl. Nurses): _____

   c) Number of full-time nursing staff: _____

5. Utilization of part-time medical staff: _____

   a) How many doctors have worked in your hospital on a part-time or affiliation basis over the last month? _____

   b) How are they paid?

      i) general income sharing

ii) fixed salaries

iii) fees directly charged to patients

iv) other (please state)_____

6.   Utilization of part-time nursing staff:

a) How many part-time nurses are on your staff (all shifts)?
(Count only those who have worked in the last 30 days)
_____

b) How many hours a week on average do they contribute?
_____

7.   What is the annual budget (total expenditures or cost) for your
hospital?
_____

8.   What percentage of these expenditures are directly related to patient
care?

_____

9.   Would you agree to the following statements?

a) There are very few restrictions on doctors' autonomy in prescribing
diagnostic tests in your hospital

         Disagree   1   2   3   4   5   very much agree
b) There are very few restrictions on doctors' autonomy in prescribing
medications in your hospital

         Disagree   1   2   3   4   5   very much agree
c) There are very few restrictions on doctors' autonomy in prescribing
therapies in your hospital

         Disagree   1   2   3   4   5   very much agree

The following is for non-HA hospitals only

10. What is the average percentage markup on direct costs related to patient
care? _____

a) medications: _____

b) doctors' time (percentage of fees payable to the hospital) :
_____

c) lab. tests: _____

d) X-rays: _____

11.   Do you run a profit or deficit in your current operations?

a) profit   b) deficit

12.   (if hospital operation is in deficit) Do you expect your deficit to rise or fall?

a) rise   b) fall

12a. Why?

_____

_____

13.   Is your hospital planning to expand?

a.Yes   b. No

13a   (if yes) In what area?

_____

Thank You Very Much for Your Assistance.

Public Survey on Medical Care, Hong Kong, November 1996

We are doing a survey for the Hong Kong Centre for Economic Research and Lingnan College Centre for Public Policy Studies on Hong Kong's medical sector. Can I talk to the head of your household?

Background:

Male   Female

Age:

Below 25 years old

26 to 35 years old

36 to 45 years old

46 to 60 years old

Over 60

What is the age of the oldest member of your household?

_____

What is the age of the youngest member of your household?

_____

How many family members do you have?

Adults_____ Children_____

Family Income

HK$15,001 to HK$30,000

HK$30,001 to HK$45,000

HK$45,001 to HK$100,000

Above HK$100,000

1a. How much do you expect to have spent on medical care, inclusive of health insurance expenditures, relative to your household income this year (percentage)? _____

1b. Does your employer provide medical insurance / benefit?

   Yes   No   I am not an employee

2. Has there been an occasion, over the last three years, in which you have had difficulty meeting unforeseen medical expenses?

   Yes   No

2a. If yes to 2, how much was needed in that year? What was your household income in that year?

   Medical Expenses_____

   Total Yearly Income_____

3a. Have you or your family used the services of a private hospital in the past 3 years?

   Yes   No

3b. Have you or your family used the services of a public hospital in the past 3 years?

   Yes   No

4. How would you rate HA hospitals relative to private hospitals?

   1: poor; 5: excellent

	Hospital Authority	Private Hospital
Value for money / Degree of satisfaction	1 2 3 4 5	1 2 3 4 5
Fast Diagnostic Services	1 2 3 4 5	1 2 3 4 5
Faster Medical Treatment (such as surgery)	1 2 3 4 5	1 2 3 4 5
Attracts Greater Trust	1 2 3 4 5	1 2 3 4 5
Environment	1 2 3 4 5	1 2 3 4 5
Nursing Care	1 2 3 4 5	1 2 3 4 5
Autonomy or choice over treatment / services	1 2 3 4 5	1 2 3 4 5
Communication between medical staff and family / patient	1 2 3 4 5	1 2 3 4 5

5. Are you willing to pay more taxes in order to get better medical services?

   Yes   No

6. Are you worried about unforeseen medical expenses?

   | 1 | 2 | 3 | 4 | 5 |

   Very much worried   Not at all worried

APPENDIX B

Cost Structure in Health Care

The Distinction between Fixed Cost and Variable Cost

The distinction in economic theory between fixed cost and variable cost, though conceptually clear at first sight, is actually very controversial. In practice, it is difficult to apply the distinctions. Walter Oi (1962) showed that much of labour costs which had long been regarded as variable are more appropriately considered as a component of overhead cost. Within the Hospital Authority, labour costs account for over 80% of total costs. If labour costs were regarded as variable, then some 90% of HA's total costs would be variable. The idea of charging patients according to marginal costs in an attempt to recover variable costs would lead to unacceptably high fees.

Despite the conceptual difficulties of defining fixed cost as distinct from variable cost, this distinction is of utmost importance in the design of a cost-recovery mechanism that is consistent with efficiency. In the health care sector, given the problem of information asymmetry between health care professionals and patients, the provision of services is very much supplier-driven. As a result, a fee-for-service setup, with fees charged and set by suppliers at levels that offer them a high profit, has been observed to drive up demand, and hence cost, excessively. In China, where hospitals are allowed to earn a markup on drugs sold, hospitals are known to oversupply drugs (Ho 1995). In France, also, evidence of supplier-driven demand is found, in the form of a significant and positive correlation between the percentage of physicians opting for their own determination of fees (for which privilege they have fewer advantages in pensions and tax treatment) and the physician density of the area (Mosse 1994). In the United States "[fee for service] may have contributed to competition between suppliers on the basis of higher quality rather than lower price, and excessive diffusion of expensive medical technologies." (OECD 1994, citing Weisbrod 1991)

It makes sense for the government to fund fixed costs and to charge users of health care services for the marginal or direct costs of the services. This way, services will be used up to the point where the marginal benefit is equal to the marginal cost. The assumption is that users are well informed of the benefit, or assuming the service providers "internalize" the benefits of the users and decide for the users. Labour should be charged at the average variable cost that would prevail under the normal or the expected rate of utilization, and charged for drugs and materials should be at cost. This way, health service providers will only recover costs and will not make a profit under normal circumstances. If they cannot increase their profit by supplying more services, they will not oversupply services.

Some of the labour costs are fixed because (1) they have to be defrayed just to maintain the running of the hospital, (2) doctors and nurses spend some of their time in administration and in research, areas which may not directly relate to the number of patients served, and (3) the medical team and the medical facilities provide the entire community an insurance value just for being available. There is not, as yet, an entirely objective way of determining how labour costs are divided between fixed and variable components.

Nevertheless, it should be noted that the utilization rate of HA hospitals averages around 81% (according to the survey conducted) while HA doctors reported an average of 82.5% of their time being spent on clinical duties. In light of the insurance value of hospital services to the entire community, and in light of these figures, we propose the following scheme of dividing up the costs:

1. All costs not directly related to the delivery of services to patients (such as cost of full-time administrators, accountants, janitors, receptionists, maintenance staff, and security staff) be treated as fixed and not chargeable to the patient; such costs should be funded directly by a transfer from the government.

2. 80% of the cost of medical staff (including therapists, technicians, and laboratory staff in charge of diagnostic services) who do not have administrative duties be deemed variable and notionally chargeable to patients. This means that patients have to pay for these costs up to the yearly threshold, but beyond the thresholds, costs are chargeable to the government.

3. Total variable costs excluding drug and diagnostic costs (which would be incurred under normal intensity of utilization) be apportioned among patients according to their use of the services in such a way that total cost recovered will cover total variable costs. Since the balance of all costs is covered by the government, each hospital will break even when the capacity is utilized to the designed, normal capacity.

4. All drugs or materials directly used on behalf of patients for clinical or diagnostic purposes be treated as variable costs and attributed to patients at cost. This way, excessive vending of drugs or materials would not occur as it did in China.

5. Charges for services in excess of the design or normal capacity be subject to a discount so as to discourage hospitals from providing services in excess of the design or normal capacity and reaping the profit from fees charged in excess of marginal costs. This may complicate the system excessively. Whether this is advisable deserves to be further studied.

APPENDIX C

Statistical Tables of Chapter 2

Table 2.1
Recurrent Budget of Hospital Authority, 1996–97

Expenditure	HK$ Million	% of Total Recurrent Expenditures
Staff cost	11,600	58.04
Staff oncosts	4,770	23.85
Sub–total	16,370	81.85
Utilities	380	1.90
Temporary staff	150	0.75
Medical supplies / instruments—drugs	1,050	5.25
Medical supplies / instruments—others	804	4.02
Repairs and maintenance	231	1.15
Hospital supplies and others	1,016	5.08
Sub–total	3,631	18.15
Total recurrent expenditure	20,001	100.00
(Minus) Income from patients	635	3.17
(Minus) Income from other sources	141	0.70
Total recurrent expenditure funded by government	19,225	96.12

Source: Hospital Authority

Appendix C

Table 2.2a
Market Share in Terms of Inpatients, 1985–95

	Government / Subvented Hospitals (inclusive of government maternity homes)	Private Hospitals
1985	84.76	15.24
1987	82.81	17.19
1989	80.69	19.31
1991	78.94	21.06
1992	79.23	20.77
1993	80.32	19.68
1994	81.44	18.56
1995	82.87	17.13
1996	83.88	16.12

Source: Hospital Authority.
Note: Figures for 1996 are provisional. Numbers in percentage.

Table 2.2b
Market Share in Terms of Inpatient Days, 1985–96

	Government / Subvented Hospitals (inclusive of government maternity homes)	Private Hospitals
1985	91.24	8.76
1987	90.73	9.27
1989	90.18	9.82
1991	90.49	9.51
1992	90.43	9.57
1993	91.18	8.82
1994	92.08	7.92
1995	92.67	7.33
1996	92.69	7.31

Source: Hospital Authority.
Note: Figures for 1996 are provisional. Numbers in percentage.

Table 2.3a
Overall Satisfaction Indicators, Public vs Private Hospitals*

Service Items	Public Sector Hospitals Score	Private Hospitals Score	Public Sector Score / Private Sector Score
Queueing time, outpatient clinic	2.524	3.589	0.7032
Queueing time, specialist clinic	2.391	3.652	0.6549
Queueing time, lab. & diagnostic tests	2.536	3.849	0.6588
Queueing time for surgery	2.331	4.031	0.5783
Attracts trust	3.375	3.726	0.9058
Environment for patients	3.283	3.938	0.8337
Nursing care	3.291	3.803	0.8654
Autonomy	2.902	3.612	0.8034
Communication with family members	2.909	3.672	0.7922
Value for money	3.775	3.312	1.1398

Source:　Public Telephone Survey (907 respondents), November 1996.
Notes:　　* Based on a telephone survey of 907 respondents. Averaged scores.
　　　　　Scoring: 1 = most unsatisfactory,　3 = fair,　5 = most satisfactory

Table 2.3b
Overall Satisfaction Indicators, Frequency of Expression of Satisfaction*

	Public Sector Hospitals Score	Private Hospitals Score	Public Sector Score / Private Sector Score #
Queueing time, Outpatient clinic	306+67+29=402	199+255+75=529	0.76 (0.59)
Queueing time, Specialist clinic	178+83+21=282	139+201+72=412	0.68 (0.57)
Queueing time, lab. & diagnostic tests	182+77+25=284	105+217+95=417	0.68 (0.57)
Queueing time for surgery	148+52+17=217	75+228+126=429	0.51 (0.47)
Attracts trust	328+288+91=707	198+337+105=640	1.10 (1.00)
Environment for patients	336+275+49=660	131+351+130=612	1.08 (1.01)
Nursing care	333+273+50=656	169+321+105=595	1.10 (1.02)
Autonomy	259+160+34=453	199+235+77=511	0.89 (0.82)
Communication with family members	269+185+38=492	178+290+86=376	0.89 (0.82)
Value for money	205+319+212=736	225+208+84=517	1.42 (0.99)

Source:　Public Telephone Survey (907 respondents), 1996.
Notes:　　# Figures in brackets indicate the ratios as calculated from a subsample of 215
　　　　　respondents who had experience using *both* private and public hospital facilities within
　　　　　the preceding three years.
　　　　　* Scores in this table are the number of respondents checking three satisfactory scores
　　　　　(Satisfaction = Satisfied + Very Good + Excellent).

Table 2.4a

Quality of Care as Perceived by Hospital Authority Doctors
(1= Do Not Agree; 5= Strongly Agree)

Statements on Quality of Care: About	"Nursing support is adequate"	"Reasonably good care is provided"	"Patients are seldom denied the most appropriate care because of a lack of resource"	"Doctors' heavy work load will not jeopardize quality"*
HA Hospitals	2.17	3.58	3.31	1.98
Private Hospitals	2.84	3.50	3.11	3.14
Ratio	0.76	1.02	1.06	0.63

Source: Doctors' Survey, November 1996 to January 1997.
Notes: * The average score here is derived by subtracting the raw average score from 5 *plus 1*
                in the question "Do you think the workload will jeopardize the quality of care?".

Table 2.4b

Quality of Care as Perceived by Private Hospital Doctors
(1 = Do Not Agree; 5 = Strongly Agree)

Statements on Quality of Care: About	"Nursing support is adequate"	"Reasonably good care is provided"	"Patients are seldom denied the most appropriate care because of a lack of resource"	"Doctors' heavy work load will not jeopardize quality"*
HA hospitals	2.46	3.61	3.49	2.06
Private hospitals	2.81	3.64	3.46	3.74
Ratio	0.87	0.99	1.04	0.55

Source: Doctors' Survey, November 1996 to January 1997.
Notes: * See notes in Table 2.4a.

Table 2.5
Those Preferring Private Hospital by Household Income

Income Category	Frequency Opting for Private Hospital	% Opting for Private Hospital	% in the Income Category
Below $15,000	90 (out of 385)	23.3	28.0
$15,001–$30,000	112 (out of 276)	40.6	37.9
$31,000–$45,000	58 (out of 103)	56.3	18.1
$45,001–$100,000	39 (out of 75)	52.0	12.1
Above $100,000	7 (out of 12)	58.0	2.2
Income not reported	25 (out of 56)	44.6	4.7
Total	321 (out of 907)	35.4	100

Source: Telephone Survey, November 1996.

Table 2.6
Willingness to Pay More Taxes to Get Better Services

Attitude to Paying More	Frequency	% of *All* Respondents
No	260 (59)	28.6 (27.4)
Yes (including those qualifying with "depending on the amount of taxes")	570 (134)	62.8 (62.3)
Invalid / missing responses	77 (22)	8.5 (10.2)
Total	907 (215)	100.0 (100.0)

Source: Telephone Survey, November 1996.

Note: Percentages do not sum to 100 because of rounding. Brackets show figures as indicated by the subsample of respondents who had experience using both private and public hospital facilities within the preceding three years.

Table 2.7

**Those Willing to Pay More Taxes for Better Services
by Household Income Categories**

Income Category	Frequency willing to pay more taxes	% willing to pay more taxes	% within income category*	% of "No" or invalid responses in income group
Below $15,000	235 (out of 346)	67.9	41.2	10.1
$15001– $30,000	177 (out of 249)	71.1	31.1	9.8
$30,001– $45,000	68 (out of 98)	69.4	11.9	4.9
$45,001–$100,000	45 (out of 74)	60.8	7.9	1.3
Over $100,000	8 (out of 12)	66.7	1.4	0
Income not reported	37 (out of 51)	72.5	6.5	20.0
Total	570 (out of 830 valid responses*)	68.5	100.0	8.5

Source: Telephone Survey, November 1996.
Notes: * Percentage of valid responses indicating a clear response of yes or no to the question.

Table 2.8

**Those Willing to Pay More Taxes for Better Services
by Age Distribution**

Age of Responding Adult in the Household	Frequency and Percentage		% of Age Group among All Who Have Reported Age
19 or below	2	(out of 2 or 100.0%)	0.2
20–29	92	(out of 139 or 66.2%)	16.2
30–39	159	(out of 280 or 57.9%)	28.9
40–49	188	(out of 280 or 67.1%)	32.8
50–59	51	(out of 91 or 56.0%)	8.9
60 and Over	73	(out of 111 or 65.8%)	13.1
Age not reported	2	(out of 4 or 50.0%)	—
Total	570 (62.8 % of all respondents)		100.0

Source: Telephone Survey, November 1996.

Table 2.9

Public Hospital Fees, 1995 and 1996

(HK$)

Service Items	1 May 95	15 November 96
Out–patient (per visit), general clinic	34	37
Out–patient (per visit), specialist clinic	40	44
Hospitalization, general ward (per day)	60	68
Hospitalization, second class (per day) (full cost recovery)	1,860	2,010
Hospitalization, first class (per day)	2,780	3,020
Emergency and accident	free	free

Source: Hospital Authority

Table 2.10

In-patients by Charges* Paid and

by Type of Hospital, 1991

(thousand patients)

Charges paid by in-patients	Government hospitals		Government-assisted hospitals		Private hospitals		Total	
Nil	3.0	(5.6)	1.4	(4.2)	4.6	(13.2)	9.0	(7.3)
$1–999	45.0	(83.7)	27.6	(80.9)	1.3	(3.7)	73.9	(60.4)
$1,000–5,999	4.7	(8.8)	4.4	(12.9)	10.4	(30.0)	19.5	(16.0)
$6,000–14,999	0.4	(0.8)	0.4	(1.2)	11.8	(34.2)	12.7	(10.3)
$15,000+	0.1	(0.3)	0.1	(0.4)	6.3	(18.1)	6.6	(5.3)
Not known	0.4	(0.8)	0.1	(0.4)	0.3	(0.8)	0.9	(0.7)
Total	57.3	(100)	34.2	(100)	34.6	(100)	122.5	(100)
Median charges	$525		$564		$6509		$701	

Source: Supplementary Enquiry via the General Household Survey, July to September 1991, Census and Statistics Department.

Note: * Charges paid by in-patients were the net charges paid for hospitalization excluding the amount subsidized by employers or insurance companies. In-patients are classified by type of hospital of last admission. (Figures in parentheses are percentage of in-patients.)

Table 2.11
Degree of Financial Difficulty in Meeting Medical Expenses

Total number of respondents	907	100.0%
Missing cases	4	0.4%
"No difficulty"	845	93.2%
"Have had difficulty"	58	6.4%
Total number of cases with financial difficulties	58	100.0%
"Having borrowed money to meet medical expenses"	34	58.6%
Not indicating borrowing	24	41.4%
Total number of cases with financial difficulties	58	100.0%
Percentage of household income spent on medical expenses		
<3%	3	5.2%
3% – 9%	2	3.4%
>9%	11	19.0%
Percentage unknown	42	72.4%

Source: Telephone Survey, November 1996.

Table 2.12
Percentage of Households Potentially at Financial Risk

Percentage of Income Spent on Health Care (%)	Number of Additional Households Potentially at Risk*	Percentage of Households Potentially at Risk if Health Care Spending Exceeds Threshold (Cumulative)
Up to 3.00	66	13.6
3.01 – 6.00	54	24.6
6.01 – 9.00	10	26.7
9.01 – 10.00	155	58.5
10.01 – 30.00	134	86.0
30.01 – 50.00	51	96.5
Over 50.00	17	100.0
Total	487	—

Source: Telephone Survey, November 1996.

Notes: * "At risk" means that the household has reported ability to afford the percentage listed. (Implying it may not have the ability to afford any percentage beyond the stated percentage.) Not all 907 respondents answered this question; 420 did not.

Table 2.13

Regression of "Not Worried Index" against Age & Income

Explanatory Variables	Regression Coefficient	t–statistic
Constant term	2.559995	16.205
Monthly household income	0.0000162479	7.149
Dummy for age at or below 29*	0.558178	2.978
Dummy for age 30 to 49 inclusive*	0.376161	2.357
Dummy for age 50 to 59 *	0.072289	1.632
Dummy for youngest member below 5	0.034008	0.315
Dummy for oldest member above 60	−0.031006	−0.273
Number of members in household	−0.008611	−0.922

Overall result: F = 9.59499; adjusted R–squared 0.06954

Source: Telephone Survey, November 1996. (Based on 805 valid observations.)

Notes: Dependent variable = 1 for most worried; = 5 for least worried.
Household income is assumed to be the middle value in the income bracket
to which the household belong. "Above $100,000" is taken to be $105,000
while "Below $15,000" is taken to be $10,000
* Coefficients are relative to the oldest group, 60+.

Table 2.14

**Domestic Households by Monthly Household Income,
Hong Kong, 1986, 1991, 1996**

Income Group	1986	1991	1996
Under $10,000	81.6%	50.2%	23.9%
$10,000–29,999	16.5%	40.9%	51.3%
$30,000–59,999	1.5	6.6%	18.0%
Over $60,000	0.4%	2.3%	6.9%
Total (households)	1,452,576 (100%)	1,582,215 (100%)	1,855,553 (100%)
Average household size	3.7	3.4	3.3
Median monthly household income	$5,160	$9,964	$17,50

Source: *1996 Population By–census: Summary Results*, 1996

Note: Domestic household is defined as a number of person(s) living together and
making common provision for essentials for living. Size refers to the number
of residents living in the domestic household.

Table 2.15a
Median Charges for Private Practitioners, 1996
(HK$)

Services	General Services (317 respondents)	Specialist Services (388 respondents)
Clinic, consultation	150	350
Clinic, simple surgery	300	600
Clinic, other surgery	1,000	2,000
Hospital doctors' fees		
1st class room	1,200	1,450
2nd class room	800	800
3rd class room	400	500
Hospital simple operation		
1st class room	2,500	2,750
2nd class room	1,500	1,900
3rd class room	1,000	1,000
Hospital minor operation		
1st class room	5,000	8,000
2nd class room	3,500	5,000
3rd class room	2,200	3,000
Hospital medium operation		
1st class room	15,000	20,000
2nd class room	9,500	13,000
3rd class room	5,000	8,000
Hospital high–level operation		
1st class room	27,500	35,000
2nd class room	15,000	20,000
3rd class room	10,000	15,000
Hospital major operation		
1st class room	70,000	60,000
2nd class room	30,000	40,000
3rd class room	20,000	25,000

Source: *Survey of Charges*, Hong Kong Medical Association, June 1996; 705 among 1995 HKMA members responded to the survey.

Table 2.15b
Actual Charges for one Private Hospital Patient, November 1996
(HK$)

Day / Total HK$	Particulars	Amount
Day 1	Treatment	5
	Laboratory	430
	Medicine / Injection	356
	Oxygen / Gas	108
1,069	Physiotherapy	170
Day 2	Treatment	654
	Laboratory	2,010
	Miscellaneous Charge	20
	Medicine / Injection	3,365
	Oxygen / Gas	216
	Physiotherapy	170
6,795	Room Charge	360
Day 3	Treatment	586
	Miscellaneous Charge	20
	Medicine / Injection	478
	Oxygen / Gas	216
	Physiotherapy	170
1,830	Room Charge	360
Day 4	Treatment	417
	Meal / Beverage	30
	Miscellaneous Charge	20
	Medicine / Injection	1,327
	Oxygen / Gas	216
2,370	Room Charge	360
Day 5	Treatment	393
	Laboratory	580
	Meal Beverage	53
	Miscellaneous Charge	20
	Medicine / Injection	3,880
	Oxygen / Gas	108
	Physiotherapy	170
	X Ray	290
5,854	Room Charge	360
Total	All Items	17,918

Source: Actual statement of account from one patient.

Table 2.16a

Doctor's Ratings of Professional Autonomy in Hong Kong's Hospitals

Doctor's Rating of Autonomy	HA Hospitals (%)	Non-HA Hospitals (%)
Very Low	4.8	1.7
Low	19.8	10.6
Neutral	36.3	29.4
High	33.9	37.2
Very High	5.2	21.1
HCE's* average rating of autonomy in diagnostic **tests**	3.75	5.00
HCE's average rating of autonomy in prescribing **medications**	3.58	4.67
HCE's average rating of autonomy in prescribing **therapies**	4.18	4.67

Source: Doctors' Survey and Hospital Administrators' Survey, December 1996.

Note: Percentages are out of valid responses (248 for HA and 180 for private hospitals; doctors from both HA and private sectors are pooled).
* HCE = Hospital Chief Executive's ratings are based on a scale of 1 to 5 with 5 being the highest in autonomy.

Table 2.16b

Professional Autonomy in Hong Kong's Hospitals

Practice Mode	Hospital Authority	Non-HA
Private practice without affiliation with any private hospital	3.28	4.18
Private practice with affiliation with a private hospital	3.25	4.21
Practice with a HA Hospital	3.11	3.49
Practice as an employee of a private hospital	2.71	3.43
Practice as an employee of a company / organization	3.00	4.00

Source: Doctors' Survey as in Table 2.16a.

Note: Average Scores of Rating by Doctors in Different Practice Modes.

Table 2.17
Reasons Cited for Preference by Frequency Cited

Reasons Cited	HA Hospital Score for Preference	Private Hospital Score for Preference
Cost is lower	409	0
Service is better	50	173
Choice over doctors	3	12
Greater confidence	24	28
Reasonable queueing time	6	88
Complete facilities	46	2

Source: Public Survey, November 1996.

Table 2.18
Attrition Rates for Workers in HA, 1995 and 1996
(%)

Type of worker	April–September 1995	October 1995–March 1996
Doctors	7.41	6.64
Nurses	11.53	9.75
Paramedics	9.43	8.85
Administrative, management, and other professionals	13.91	11.43
Supporting	9.03	6.64

Source: *Ming Pao*, 6 June 96.

Bibliography

1. Aaron, Henry (1994). "Issues Every Plan to Reform Health Care Financing Must Confront," *Journal of Economic Perspectives* 8, No. 3 (Summer): 31–43.

2. Abel-Smith, Brian (1994). *Introduction to Health: Policy, Planning, and Financing*. London: Longman.

3. Arnett, Jerome C., Jr. (1996). "Ontario's Health Care: A Pox on Doctors and Patients," *The Asian Wall Street Journal* (3 October): 8.

4. Barr, Nicholas (1992). "Economic Theory and the Welfare State: a survey and interpretation," *Journal of Economic Literature* (June): 749–755; 779–798.

5. Baumol, William J. and David F. Bradford (1970). "Optimal Departures from Marginal Cost Pricing," *American Economic Review* 60(3) (June): 265–83.

6. Coalition of Groups Concerned about Medical Care (1995). *Community Green Paper on Health Care Services*.

7. Glennerster, Howard and Manos Matsaganis (1992). *The English and Swedish Health Care Reforms*. London: London School of Economics: The Welfare State Programme Discussion Paper WSP/79.

8. Hay, Joel W. (1992). *Health Care in Hong Kong*. Hong Kong: Chinese University Press for Hong Kong Centre for Economic Research.

9. Ho, Lok Sang (1995). "Market Reform and China's Health Care System," *Social Sciences and Medicine* 41, No. 8 (October).

10. Kwa, Soon Bee (1996). "Health Care Financing — The Singapore Model," speech delivered at the International Health Federation Pan Regional Conference / Hong Kong Hospital Authority Convention.

11. Laaser, U, E. J. Roccella, J. B. Rosenfeld, H. Wenzel (1990) (eds). *Costs and Benefits in Health Care and Prevention*. Berlin: Springer-Verlag.

12. Lamm, Richard D. (1994). "The Ethics of Excess," *Hastings Center Report* 24, No. 6: 14.

13. McPhee, Debra (1995). "Health Care in the United States: The Battle of Reform," *Journal of Health and Social Policy* 7: pp. 69–86.

14. Morreim, E. Harrvi (1995). *Balancing Act: The New Medical Ethics of Medicine's New Economics.* Washington, D.C.: Georgetown University Press.

15. Mosse, Ph. R. (1994). "Towards a Professional Rationalization: Lessons from the French Health Care System," *American Journal of Economics and Sociology* 53, No. 2 (April): 129–146.

16. OECD (1994) *The Reform of the Health Care Systems: A Review of Seventeen OECD Countries.* Paris: OECD (Health Policy Studies No. 5)

17. Oi, Walter (1962). "Labour as a Quasi Fixed Factor," *Journal of Political Economy 70: 538–555.*

18. Oxley, Howard and Maitland MacFarlan (1994). *Health Care Reform: Controlling Spending and Increasing Efficiency.* Paris: OECD.

19. Phua, Kai Hong (1991). *Privatization and Restructuring of Health Services in Singapore.* Singapore: The Institute of Policy Studies, Times Academic Press.

20. Stoline, Anne M. and Jonathan P. Weiner (1993). *The New Medical Marketplace: A Physician's Guide to the Health Care System in the 1990s.* Baltimore: Johns Hopkins University Press.

21. Weisbrod, B. (1991). "Health Care Quadrilemma: an Essay on Technological Change, Insurance, Quality of Care and Cost Containment," *Journal of Economic Literature,* XXIX (June).

Index

A

accessibility (see also financial)
22–23, 34, 40, 55–56, 58, 63,
85, 93–94, 97, 105
adverse selection 49–50, 72, 77
Advertising 102
ageing 5, 7, 12, 17, 20, 40, 45, 48
Alan Maynard 68
Alternative Models (health care) 99
attrition rate 40, 133
autonomy 22–23, 29, 32, 39–41,
73–78, 94–97, 112
Professional Autonomy in
Hospitals 132

B

budget 4, 20, 31, 34–35, 37–41, 45,
47, 55–56, 59, 85, 94–95, 97,
101, 112, 121
budget cap 75, 78, 80, 83, 87
burden 32–37, 55–58, 93–105

C

capping (see also budget cap) 64
Charges and Fees
Actual Charges for one Private
Hospital Patient 131
Fees of Primary Care Services
104
In-patients by Type of Hospital
127
Median Charges for Private
Practitioners 130
Public Hospital Fees 127
Choice and Autonomy 73
Choice for Better Services (see also
freedom of choice) 87, 89

consumption efficiency 37
copayment 72
Cost (see marginal cost and variable
cost)
cost containment 80, 92

D

defensive medicine 50, 73, 76, 93
Demographics (see also ageing
Ageing and Demographic Trends
in Hong Kong 5
demographic pressure 48
Death Rates in Hospitals 4
mortality rate 10
Distributional Aspects of Health
Policy 51
Doctors
Average Working Hours 6
Doctors in Public vs Private
Hospitals 6, 124
Perception of Impact of Resource
Constraint 6
Quality of Care, as Perceived by
124
Ratings Professional Autonomy
132

E

economic dimensions of health care
8
efficiency wage 67–68
Efficient Production of Health 47
Evaluative Framework 21

F

financial accessibility 21, 23, 28, 32,
40, 55–56, 64, 96, 105

Are the Poor Denied Needed
    Services 28
Financial Burden 32, 62
Financial Difficulty in Meeting
    Medical Expenses 128
Financial Problems & Risks 32, 63
    Difficulty in Meeting Medical
        Expenses 128
    Households Potentially at
        Financial Risk 128
financial risk 63
fixed cost 58, 86, 7–118
freedom of choice 22, 29, 38, 61,
    64, 83, 94

G

global budget cap 78–79

H

health care expenditures 9–10, 33,
    50–51, 78–79, 84, 87–88,
    92–93, 102
    Expenditures Relative to GDP 8,
        10
    Recurrent Budget of Hospital
        Authority 121
    Yearly Health Spending Limits for
        Household 86
health care system 5, 7, 9–10, 19,
    22–24, 26, 28–29, 35, 37, 40,
    61, 63, 67, 75, 80, 83, 85, 89,
    100, 104, 108, 111
health policy 8, 43, 51–52, 55, 85
HMO 19–20, 41, 66–68, 91, 93
Hospital Authority (HA) 1–4, 9, 13,
    15–16, 18–19, 28, 30, 32,
    36–40, 67, 81, 88, 90, 96–97,
    104, 107, 117, 121, 124, 127
    Attrition Rates for Workers 133
    Bed Supply & Activities 16
    Death Rates in HA Hospitals 4
    Fees of Primary Care Services 104
    Quality of Care as Perceived by
        HA Doctors 124
    Recurrent Budget 121

Hospital Beds
    Bed Adequacy vs Bed Occupancy
        14
    Hospital Bed Supply & Activities
        16
Hospital Services Department 2, 41
Hospitalization Rates 11, 12–13
Hospitals, Public vs Private
    Average Working Hours 6
    In-patients by Charges 127
    Market Share (Inpatient Days)
        122
    Market Share (Inpatients) 122
    Overall Satisfaction 123
    Perception of Impact of Resource
        Constraint 6
    Preferring Private Hospital by
        Household Income 125
    Professional Autonomy 132
    Public Hospital Fees 127
    Quality of Care 124
    Reasons Cited for Preference
        133
Household Characteristics
    household behaviour 47
    Household Income 125, 126, 129
    Potentially at Financial Risk 30,
        128
    Preferring Private Hospital 125
    Willing to Pay More Taxes for
        Better Services 126
    Yearly Health Spending Limits
        86
household production 43
Human Capital Investment Problem
    69

I

Impact of the Medisave Plan of
    Singapore 100
income of household 29–31, 33–34,
    115
information asymmetry 48, 117
information cost 48, 61, 65, 69, 77,
    80

insurance 15, 17, 19, 33–34, 47,
    49–50, 52, 56–57, 59, 61–63,
    65–67, 70–73, 77, 79, 93–97,
    99, 101, 115, 118, 127
  Decline in Job-related Health
    Insurance in the U.S. 51
  deductible 49, 62, 72, 90
  Premiums of Blue Cross Medical
    Insurance 73
  private 83, 89–90
International Comparison
  Health Care Expenditures
    Relative to GDP 8

J

Joel Hay 104

L

least burden 22, 36, 62

M

malpractice compensation 50–51,
    72–73, 76, 83, 92–94
marginal cost 36–37, 58–59, 62, 77,
    86–87, 90–91, 94, 100–101,
    117–119
medical expenses 31, 34, 64, 71,
    115–116, 128
Medical Ombudsman 103
Medisave 64, 71–72, 84, 99–100
Medishield 71–72, 84, 99
moral hazard 48–49, 68–71, 78, 84,
    87, 94
  Moral Hazard Problem 62, 65
mortality rate 10

N

National Health Plan of Singapore
    71

O

OECD 5, 9, 101, 118
Ombudsman, Medical 103
optimal allocation of resources 21

P

Policy Options (see also health
    policy; and Recommendations)
    8–9, 53, 59, 61–63
  Autonomy 75–77
  Burden 78–80
  Choice 75–77, 94
  Hay's model 99
  Insurance (private) 89–90
  Insurance (universal) 84–89,
    102–106
  models (see Hay, Singapore,
    Sweden)
  Moral Hazards 62, 65
  Risk Management 71–73
  Singapore 99–101
  Sweden 101–102
Preferring Private Hospital by
    Household Income 125, 133
Premiums of Blue Cross Medical
    Insurance 73
PRG 38, 81, 95, 97
primary care 3, 20, 104
principal–agent problem 49, 61,
    65–66, 69, 80, 83, 97
Principles in Health Policy 45, 47,
    49, 51, 53, 55, 57, 59, 63
Private Health Care Provider's Role
    90
private health insurance 83, 89–90
Production Efficiency and
    Consumption Efficiency 32,
    36, 37, 50
professional autonomy 39, 83,
    94–95, 109
Public Debate on Burden 35
public hospital fees 29

Q

Quality, Better (than now) 89
quality-adjusted life years (QALY)
    54
quality of care 7, 26, 67, 96, 110,
    124

quality of service 20, 22, 23, 31, 40, 63, 66, 74, 79, 88, 124

R

Rates
   Attrition Rates for Workers in HA, 1995 and 1996 133
   Death Rates in 10 Major Hospital Authority Hospitals 4
   Hospitalization Rates, Hong Kong, 1989–95 11
   mortality rate 10
   Utilization Rates and Resource Input 12
Recommendations (see also Policy Options) 2, 8, 83–98
Resources
   Allocation of 21, 38
   Growth of Resource Input 13
   input 37–38
   Perception of Impact of Resource Constraint 6
   Utilization Rates and Resource Input 12
Risk (see Financial Problems)
   Not Worried Index 129
   Potentially at Financial Risk 63, 128
   risk management 61, 70–71, 78
   risk pooling 71

S

Satisfaction
   Frequency of Expression of Satisfaction 123
   Public vs Private Hospitals 123

Scott Report 2
Singapore
   Impact of the Medisave Plan 100
   Medishield 71–72, 84, 99
Singapore Model 71, 99
supply-side moral hazard 67–68, 87, 91
Sweden 101–103
System (health) under Stress 9

T

taxes 7, 15, 17, 19–20, 26–28, 35–36, 41, 47, 55, 57–58, 62, 76, 78–79, 85, 87, 116, 126
Tax-paid Doctors as Patient Advocates 91
trade-off 21–23, 54–55, 83, 93, 96–97

U

United States
   Decline in Job-related Health Insurance Coverage 51
Universal Excess Burden Health Insurance Plan 8, 101
   UEBHIP 9, 84–85, 88–90, 97, 99
   Universal Insurance for All 84
User Charges 85
   user pays principle 63
utilization rate 1, 12, 25, 69, 118

V

value of health 43
value of life 60
variable cost 33, 36–37, 60, 86, 93, 117–119

About the Author

Lok Sang Ho is Professor of Economics and Director of the Centre for Public Policy Studies of Lingnan College, Hong Kong. He is also an Honorary Research Fellow of the Hong Kong Institute of Asian Pacific Studies at The Chinese University of Hong Kong. A graduate of The University of Hong Kong and holding a doctorate from the University of Toronto, Professor Ho is interested in a wide range of public policy areas including health, social security, labour, social economics, housing, transportation, macroeconomic policy, and land economics. Currently he is Managing Editor of *Pacific Economic Review*.

The Hong Kong Economic Policy Studies Series

Titles	Authors
Hong Kong and the Region	
❏ The Political Economy of Laissez Faire	Yue-Chim Richard WONG
❏ Hong Kong and South China: The Economic Synergy	Yun-Wing SUNG
❏ Inflation in Hong Kong	Alan K. F. SIU
❏ Trade and Investment: Mainland China, Hong Kong and Taiwan	K. C. FUNG
❏ Tourism and the Hong Kong Economy	Kai-Sun KWONG
❏ Economic Relations between Hong Kong and the Pacific Community	Yiu-Kwan FAN
Money and Finance	
❏ The Monetary System of Hong Kong	Y. F. LUK
❏ The Linked Exchange Rate System	Yum-Keung KWAN Francis T. LUI
❏ Hong Kong as an International Financial Centre: Evolution, Prospects and Policies	Y. C. JAO
❏ Corporate Governance: Listed Companies in Hong Kong	Richard Yan-Ki HO Stephen Y. L. CHEUNG
❏ Institutional Development of the Insurance Industry	Ben T. YU
Infrastructure and Industry	
❏ Technology and Industry	Kai-Sun KWONG
❏ Competition Policy and the Regulation of Business	Leonard K. CHENG Changqi WU
❏ Telecom Policy and Digital Convergence	Milton MUELLER
❏ Port Facilities and Container Handling Services	Leonard K. CHENG Yue-Chim Richard WONG

Titles	Authors
❏ Efficient Transport Policy	Timothy D. HAU Stephen CHING
❏ Competition in Energy	Pun-Lee LAM
❏ Privatizing Water and Sewage Services	Pun-Lee LAM Yue-Cheong CHAN

Immigration and Human Resources

❏ Labour Market in a Dynamic Economy	Wing SUEN William CHAN
❏ Immigration and the Economy of Hong Kong	Kit Chun LAM Pak Wai LIU
❏ Youth, Society and the Economy	Rosanna WONG Paul CHAN

Housing and Land

❏ The Private Residential Market	Alan K. F. SIU
❏ On Privatizing Public Housing	Yue-Chim Richard WONG
❏ Housing Policy for the 21st Century: Homes for All	Rosanna WONG
❏ Financial and Property Markets: Interactions Between the Mainland and Hong Kong	Pui-King LAU
❏ Town Planning in Hong Kong: A Critical Review	Lawrence Wai-Chung LAI

Social Issues

❏ Retirement Protection: A Plan for Hong Kong	Francis T. LUI
❏ Income Inequality and Economic Development	Hon-Kwong LUI
❏ Health Care Delivery and Financing: A Model for Reform	Lok Sang HO
❏ Economics of Crime and Punishment	Siu Fai LEUNG